W9-CKT-844

Praise for *Implementing the Evidence-Based Practice (EBP) Competencies in Healthcare*

"This book fills a significant gap in the literature and emphasizes the importance of evidence-based practice in expert clinical practice. The authors are champions in the EBP field, and all who read this book will find it empowering. I am excited to see a body of knowledge organized in one book that will truly impact how EBP can be effectively implemented throughout healthcare systems locally and globally. Congratulations on such a landmark publication!"

–Marilyn Hockenberry, PhD, RN-PPCNP-BC, FAAN
Bessie Baker Professor of Nursing, Professor of Pediatrics
Associate Dean for Research Affairs
Duke University School of Nursing
Chair, Duke Institutional Review Board

"In our fast-paced healthcare environment, implementing evidence into practice is even more critical to improve outcomes. As leaders, we need to embrace evidence-based practice and are responsible for building the culture of inquiry that will move healthcare forward. This book covers the practical, step-by-step guidelines to implement such a culture. Melnyk, Gallagher-Ford, and Fineout-Overholt do an excellent job of providing the competencies necessary to implement and sustain an evidence-based practice culture."

–Jeanine M. Rundquist, DNP, RN, NEA-BC
Director of Performance, Practice and Innovation and Magnet Program Director
Children's Hospital Colorado

"Competence in evidence-based practice (EBP) is key to the success of RNs and APNs in implementing, sustaining, and disseminating best practices. These research-based EBP competences are presented as a user-friendly, easy-to-implement tool that provides structure and support for nursing leaders in building a culture of EBP that will move their organization forward."

–Penelope Gorsuch, DNP, RN, ACNP-BC, CCNS, NEA-BC, CCRN-K
Dean, USAF School of Aerospace Medicine*
*This should not be viewed as an official endorsement by the School of Aerospace Medicine or the United States Air Force

"A practical, much-needed guide for nurses and leaders in clinical settings to understand, apply, and sustain evidence-based practices that promote quality and safety and patient engagement. This resource embraces the complexity of today's healthcare systems and skillfully provides busy clinicians with important steps in the EBP process, related competencies, strategies to promote the competencies, and assessment indicators. Real-world examples—along with content for shared governance, policy and procedure committees, and educators—make the steps meaningful and manageable."

–Sharon Tucker, PhD, RN, PMHCNS-BC, FAAN
Robert Wood Johnson Executive Nurse Fellow Alumna (2007-10)
Director, Nursing Research, Evidence-Based Practice & Quality, Department of Nursing Services and Patient Care, University of Iowa Hospitals & Clinics

Also by Bernadette Mazurek Melnyk and Ellen Fineout-Overholt,
Implementing Evidence-Based Practice: Real-Life Success Stories

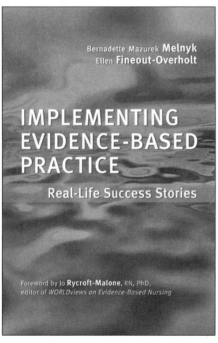

ISBN: 9781935476689

Evidence-based practice has emerged as one of the most important healthcare movements of the 21st century. But the challenge for many nurses is incorporating evidence-based practice in their daily routine and sustaining it. In *Implementing Evidence-Based Practice: Real-Life Success Stories,* real clinicians share their experiences with paradigm shifts to EBP, implementation of the EBP process to change practice and improve patient outcomes, personal experiences with evidence-based care, and transforming systems to an EBP culture.

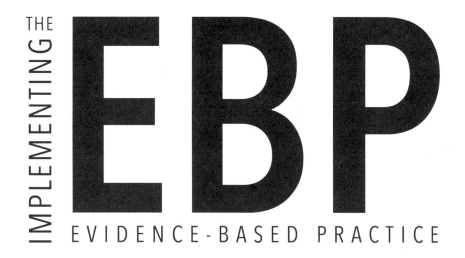

IMPLEMENTING THE EBP
EVIDENCE-BASED PRACTICE

COMPETENCIES IN HEALTHCARE

A PRACTICAL GUIDE FOR IMPROVING QUALITY, SAFETY, AND OUTCOMES

BERNADETTE MAZUREK MELNYK, PHD, RN, CPNP/PMHNP, FAANP, FNAP, FAAN

LYNN GALLAGHER-FORD, PHD, RN, DPFNAP, NE-BC

ELLEN FINEOUT-OVERHOLT, PHD, RN, FNAP, FAAN

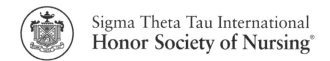

Sigma Theta Tau International
Honor Society of Nursing®

The Honor Society of Nursing, Sigma Theta Tau International (STTI) is a nonprofit organization founded in 1922 whose mission is to support the learning, knowledge, and professional development of nurses committed to making a difference in health worldwide. Members include practicing nurses, instructors, researchers, policymakers, entrepreneurs, and others. STTI has more than 500 chapters located at more than 700 institutions of higher education throughout Armenia, Australia, Botswana, Brazil, Canada, Colombia, England, Ghana, Hong Kong, Japan, Kenya, Lebanon, Malawi, Mexico, the Netherlands, Pakistan, Portugal, Singapore, South Africa, South Korea, Swaziland, Sweden, Taiwan, Tanzania, Thailand, the United Kingdom, and the United States of America. More information about STTI can be found online at www.nursingsociety.org.

Sigma Theta Tau International
550 West North Street
Indianapolis, IN, USA 46202

To order additional books, buy in bulk, or order for corporate use, contact Nursing Knowledge International at 888.NKI.4YOU (888.654.4968/US and Canada) or +1.317.634.8171 (outside US and Canada).

To request a review copy for course adoption, email solutions@nursingknowledge.org or call 888.NKI.4YOU (888.654.4968/US and Canada) or +1.317.634.8171 (outside US and Canada).

To request author information, or for speaker or other media requests, contact Marketing, Honor Society of Nursing, Sigma Theta Tau International at 888.634.7575 (US and Canada) or +1.317.634.8171 (outside US and Canada).

ISBN:	9781940446424
EPUB ISBN:	9781940446431
PDF ISBN:	9781940446448
MOBI ISBN:	9781940446455

Library of Congress Cataloging-in-Publication data

Names: Melnyk, Bernadette Mazurek, author. | Gallagher-Ford, Lynn, 1957- , author. | Fineout-Overholt, Ellen, author. | Sigma Theta Tau International, issuing body.
Title: Implementing the evidence-based practice (EBP) competencies in healthcare : a practical guide for improving quality, safety, and outcomes / Bernadette Mazurek Melnyk, Lynn Gallagher-Ford, Ellen Fineout-Overholt.
Description: Indianapolis, IN : Sigma Theta Tau International, [2016]
Identifiers: LCCN 2016014469 (print) | LCCN 2016015187 (ebook) | ISBN 9781940446424 (print : alk. paper) | ISBN 9781940446431 (epub) | ISBN 9781940446448 (pdf) | ISBN 9781940446455 (mobi) | ISBN 9781940446431 (Epub) | ISBN 9781940446448 (Pdf) | ISBN 9781940446455 (Mobi)
Subjects: | MESH: Evidence-Based Nursing | Clinical Competence | Nursing Care | Quality of Health Care
Classification: LCC RT42 (print) | LCC RT42 (ebook) | NLM WY 100.7 | DDC 610.73--dc23
LC record available at https://lccn.loc.gov/2016014469

First Printing, 2016

Publisher: Dustin Sullivan
Acquisitions Editor: Emily Hatch
Editorial Coordinator: Paula Jeffers
Cover Designer: Rebecca Batchelor
Interior Design/Page Layout: Rebecca Batchelor

Principal Book Editor: Carla Hall
Development and Project Editor: Rebecca Senninger
Copy Editor: Teresa Artman
Proofreader: Todd Lothery
Indexer: Larry Sweazy

DEDICATIONS

I dedicate this book to my loving family, John, Kaylin, Angela, and Megan, who continue to support me to follow my dreams and passions, along with all of the Advancing Research and Clinical practice through close Collaboration (ARCC) evidence-based practice mentors throughout the United States and world who ignite a spirit of inquiry in their colleagues and dedicate their careers to enhancing healthcare quality and outcomes through EBP.

—*Bernadette Mazurek Melnyk*

I dedicate this book to my husband, Jeff, who always encourages me to pursue my dreams and who has always believed in me more than I believed in myself. He is brilliant, kind, and fun . . . and he loves me more than I deserve. He has been, and continues to be, the best thing in my life.

—*Lynn Gallagher-Ford*

Most affectionately, I dedicate this book to my family, Wayne, Rachael, and Ruth, who graciously sacrifice so that I may engage in these works. They are my soul. I also dedicate this book to Megan Folmar Jennings, BSN, RN, and Ben Behnke, BSN, RN, two fine examples of emerging leaders who are committed to the lived experience of EBP. I would let them be my nurse anytime! Finally, I dedicate this book to the 14 graduates of the first EBP graduate certificate program who are pushing the envelope every day where they practice. Their tenacity, courage, and wisdom are central to the reformation we need in healthcare.

—*Ellen Fineout-Overholt*

ACKNOWLEDGMENTS

I would like to thank and acknowledge my two terrific friends and colleagues who edited and wrote this book with me: Lynn Gallagher-Ford and Ellen Fineout-Overholt. Their expertise in evidence-based practice (EBP) is unmatched, and it is always exciting to dream about and execute the next innovations and advancements in EBP together with them. We are fortunate to be able to continue our passion for and collaborative initiatives in EBP together to accomplish one of our big dreams—that by 2025, every clinician in the world will have EBP in their DNA. I also want to thank and acknowledge our entire team in the Center for Transdisciplinary Evidence-based Practice (CTEP) at The Ohio State University College of Nursing, especially Bindu Koshy Thomas, Lynn Ellingsworth, Susan Potter, and Cindy Zellefrow, who are the wind beneath Lynn's and my wings. In addition, I am thankful to Mary Nash and Jackie Buck at The Ohio State University Wexner Medical Center and Linda Stoverock, Cathleen Opperman, and Cheryl Boyd at Nationwide Children's Hospital, who have all been terrific academic-practice partners in working together with our CTEP team to create ideal EBP practice environments and cultures. Special acknowledgement also is given to all the Advancing Research and Clinical practice through close Collaboration (ARCC) model EBP mentors affiliated with our CTEP and the other five experts who served on the national expert panel for the first phase of consensus validation for the EBP competencies, including Karen Balakas, Anna Gawlinski, Marilyn Hockenberry, Rona Levin, and Teri Wurmser. It's all about the dream and the TEAM *because Together, Everyone Accomplishes More.*

—*Bernadette Mazurek Melnyk*

On behalf of myself and countless other clinicians who are passionate about EBP, I would like to acknowledge Bernadette Mazurek Melnyk for her passionate and relentless leadership in the field of evidence-based practice. Working with Bern is the most exhilarating, inspiring, rewarding "job" anyone could ever imagine. Whatever your dream is, she will encourage you to dream bigger and in brighter colors . . . and then she will be your biggest fan! The opportunity to work with this remarkable woman has been a gift to me, and I am humbled to be able to be a part of the legacy she has built and continues to grow. I would be remiss if I also did not give tremendous credit to my colleagues at the Center for

Transdisciplinary Evidence-based Practice at The Ohio State University College of Nursing. Our team is simply amazing, and what we have accomplished is absolutely the product of synergy and mutual respect for each other's talents and contributions. It is a privilege to work alongside these women every day. Finally, I would like to acknowledge the EBP champions whom I have come to know, not only through our EBP mentor programs, but also those who are out there passionately working every day to figure out how to make EBP a reality in their organizations. I am inspired by your passion, your vision, your courage, and your fortitude as you forge paths to evidence-based practice in spite of the barriers and obstacles! Carry on colleagues—together, we are changing the world!

—*Lynn Gallagher-Ford*

Thank you to Bern and Lynn for their commitment to advancing evidence-based practice and the opportunity to contribute to this important work. These EBP competencies are yet one more step toward realizing the dream of the EBP paradigm as *the* paradigm for healthcare. Thank you to my co-contributors, Tracy Brewer, Joanne Cleary-Holdforth, Tami Hartzell, Pamela Lake, Lisa Long, Tina Magers, and Dónal O'Mathúna. You are the best! Thank you to my colleagues at University of Texas at Tyler College of Nursing & Health Sciences, who have a wonderful way of fostering growth through strength. I am blessed to work with you. I so appreciate Drs. Barb Haas, Pam Martin, Gloria Duke, Danita Alfred, and Susan Yarbrough, who have encouraged me to reach new heights. Thank you to the One who loves me and sustains me with His strength. Finally, I extend my sincere appreciation to the emerging nurse leaders at the bedside, who I believe will be the change we need in healthcare. Thank you for tirelessly continuing to challenge the status quo so that healthcare improves for all of us.

—*Ellen Fineout-Overholt*

ABOUT THE AUTHORS

BERNADETTE MAZUREK MELNYK, PhD, RN, CPNP/PMHNP, FAANP, FNAP, FAAN

Bernadette Melnyk is Associate Vice President for Health Promotion, University Chief Wellness Officer, and Professor and Dean of the College of Nursing at The Ohio State University. She also is Professor of Pediatrics and Professor of Psychiatry at Ohio State's College of Medicine. Melnyk earned her bachelor of science in nursing degree from West Virginia University; her master of science in nursing, specializing in nursing care of children as a pediatric nurse practitioner, from the University of Pittsburgh; and her PhD in clinical research from the University of Rochester, where she also completed her post-master's certificate as a psychiatric mental health nurse practitioner. She is a nationally and internationally recognized expert in evidence-based practice, intervention research, child and adolescent mental health, and health and wellness and is a frequent keynote speaker at national and international conferences on these topics. Melnyk has consulted with numerous healthcare systems and colleges throughout the United States and world on how to improve quality of care and patient outcomes through implementing and sustaining evidence-based practice. She has received more than $19 million in sponsored funding from federal agencies as principal investigator and has more than 280 publications. Melnyk is co-editor of four books: *Evidence-Based Practice in Nursing & Healthcare: A Guide to Best Practice*; *Implementing Evidence-Based Practice: Real-Life Success Stories*; *A Practical Guide to Child and Adolescent Mental Health Screening, Early Intervention, and Health Promotion* (2nd ed.); and *Intervention Research: Designing, Conducting, Analyzing and Funding*. Melnyk is an elected Fellow of the National Academy of Medicine, the American Academy of Nursing, the National Academies of Practice, and the American Association of Nurse Practitioners. She served a 4-year term on the 16-member United States Preventive Services Task Force and currently serves as a member of the National Quality Forum (NQF) Behavioral Health Standing Committee and the National Institutes of Health National Advisory Council for Nursing Research. Melnyk is also Editor of the journal *Worldviews on Evidence-Based Nursing* and is a board member of U.S. Healthiest, the National Guideline Clearinghouse, and the National Quality Measures Clearinghouse.

Melnyk has received numerous national and international awards, including the Audrey Hepburn Award, Mary Tolle Wright Excellence in Leadership Award, and International Nurse Researcher Hall of Fame Award from Sigma Theta Tau International; the Jessie Scott Award from the American Nurses Association for the improvement of healthcare quality through the integration of research, education, and practice; the 2012 Midwest Nursing Research Society Senior Scientist award; the NIH/National Institute of Nursing Research inaugural director's lectureship award; and the National Organization of Nurse Practitioner Faculties Lifetime Achievement Award. She also has been recognized twice as an Edge Runner by the American Academy of Nursing for founding and directing the National Association of Pediatric Nurse Practitioners KySS child and adolescent mental health program and her COPE Program for parents of preterm infants.

Melnyk recently founded the National Interprofessional Education and Practice Collaborative to advance the DHHS Million Hearts initiative to prevent 1 million heart attacks and strokes by 2017. She also founded and is serving as the first President of the National Consortium for Building Healthy Academic Communities, a collaborative organization to improve population health in U.S. institutions of higher learning.

LYNN GALLAGHER-FORD, PHD, RN, DPFNAP, NE-BC

Lynn Gallagher-Ford is Director of the Center for Transdisciplinary Evidence-based Practice (CTEP) and Clinical Associate Professor in the College of Nursing at The Ohio State University. Gallagher-Ford earned her bachelor of science in nursing degree from Binghamton University, her master of science degree with a specialization in nursing administration from Widener University, her postgraduate certificate in nursing administration from Villanova University, and her PhD from Widener University. Gallagher-Ford is nationally certified as a nurse executive. Her clinical background in maternal-child health and nursing administration spanned 28 years; she served in a variety of roles that ranged from bedside clinician to Chief Nursing Officer. Gallagher-Ford has extensive experience and expertise in teaching and implementing evidence-based practice (EBP) in real-world clinical settings. Most recently, she has been an integral part of EBP centers at two large universities, where her work has been dedicated to research, education, and consultation focused on development, promotion, implementation, and sustainability of EBP in academic and clinical settings. In her current role as director of CTEP, she leads a world renowned, groundbreaking enterprise that generates and disseminates cutting-edge research about EBP, developing and delivering innovative programs and resources to promote effective integration and sustainability of EBP in clinical and academic settings to improve healthcare quality and patient and family outcomes. Gallagher-Ford is active as a consultant, facilitator, panelist, and keynote presenter at national and international conferences and education programs.

She is co-author of three recent studies conducted with Bernadette Melnyk that have dramatically impacted the current body of knowledge about EBP and influenced strategic imperatives to address new challenges: a national survey of nurse executives that assessed current realities related to organizational priorities, EBP attributes and investment, benchmark metrics, and outcomes; a Delphi study that established essential EBP competencies for practicing registered nurses and advanced practice nurses; and a survey of U.S. nurses that revealed an updated assessment of the state of EBP.

Gallagher-Ford was a lead author in the *American Journal of Nursing* EBP series, which received the Sigma Theta Tau International Publication Award for 2011. She is editor of the column "Implementing and Sustaining EBP in Real World Healthcare Settings" in *Worldviews on Evidence-Based Nursing,* which features best evidence-based strategies and innovative ideas on how to promote and sustain evidence-based practices and cultures in clinical organizations. Gallagher-Ford was inducted into the Nursing Academy of the National Academies of Practice as a Distinguished Practitioner and Fellow in 2013.

ELLEN FINEOUT-OVERHOLT, PHD, RN, FNAP, FAAN

Ellen Fineout-Overholt is a nationally and internationally recognized nursing leader, educator, and promoter of evidence-based practice (EBP), innovation, and leadership. She earned her PhD in clinical research from the University of Rochester in Rochester, New York; her master of science in cardiovascular nursing from the University of Alabama in Birmingham, Alabama; and her bachelor of science in nursing degree from the University of Texas Medical Branch in Galveston, Texas. Fineout-Overholt is the Mary Coulter Dowdy Distinguished Nursing Professor in the College of Nursing & Health Sciences at the University of Texas at Tyler. In this role, she realizes her passion for fostering inquiry and wonder in learners, whether they are novices or experts. She teaches and mentors undergraduate, graduate, and doctoral students in EBP and partners with community healthcare systems to advance EBP as the lived experience of every healthcare provider and patient.

As Dean of the Frank S. Groner Endowed Memorial School of Professional Studies at East Texas Baptist University and Clinical Professor and Director of the Center for the Advancement of Evidence-Based Practice at Arizona State University (ASU), she worked with faculty and students to revise curriculum to meet the national mandate for inclusion of EBP in health professions education as well as with community partners to implement EBP. During her tenure at ASU, she and her team fostered the growth of more than 300 EBP mentors, who are transforming healthcare across the globe. She also developed the first graduate certificate in EBP in the United States, which graduated 14 Expert EBP Mentors—4 of whom are contributors to this book. Her career has been devoted to building a critical mass of young leaders in nursing who will advance EBP and thereby transform healthcare. To that end, Fineout-Overholt led a team of EBP experts in writing the award-winning, widely acclaimed "EBP Step-by-Step Series" in the *American Journal of Nursing,* which is designed to demystify the EBP paradigm and process for point-of-care clinicians. She has been instrumental in the ongoing development of the Melnyk & Fineout-Overholt Advancing Research & Clinical practice through close Collaboration (ARCC) model that guides implementation of EBP in the service sector. Out of her commitment to the paradigm shift to EBP as the foundation for healthcare education, she co-edited the first "Teaching EBP" column in *Worldviews on Evidence-Based Nursing.* In addition, she developed the Fineout-Overholt & Melnyk ARCC-E model that guides integration of EBP into academic curricula. Fineout-Overholt is co-author with Melnyk of the bestselling, award-winning book *Evidence-Based Practice in Nursing & Healthcare: A Guide to Best Practice,* now in its third edition, as well as *Implementing Evidence-Based*

Practice: Real-Life Success Stories, which offers examples about how, when, where, who, and why EBP is so important to healthcare. Throughout her career, Fineout-Overholt has intentionally focused on a grassroots approach to advancing EBP. She has published extensively on EBP and has received numerous honors in recognition of her contributions to nursing, including election as a Fellow of the American Academy of Nursing and the National Academies of Practice. She serves on the editorial boards of *Worldviews on Evidence-Based Nursing* and *Research and Theory for Nursing Practice.*

CONTRIBUTING AUTHORS

Cheryl Boyd, PhD, RN, NE-BC, WHNP-BC, CNS, is Director of Professional Development for Nationwide Children's Hospital in Columbus, Ohio. She is board certified as a nurse executive and as a women's health nurse practitioner. She worked in nurse practitioner and program director positions in Tennessee with rural and urban underserved adolescent and adult patient populations. Boyd has 10 years of faculty and department head experience in undergraduate nursing programs. At The Ohio State University Medical Center (OSUMC), she was the Director of the Center for Nursing Excellence overseeing the Magnet Recognition Program®, nursing quality, nursing research, and professional development programs. In her current position, she oversees the provision of clinical education and staff development at Nationwide Children's Hospital. In addition to leading the Patient/Family Policy Committee for the past 7 years, she recently successfully completed leadership of a third Magnet Recognition Program designation. (Chapter 12)

Tracy Brewer, DNP, RNC-OB, CLC, is an Associate Professor at Wright State University College of Nursing & Health in Dayton, Ohio. She received her doctor of nursing practice in educational leadership from Case Western Reserve University, her master of nursing in education from Drexel University, and her bachelor of science in nursing from Miami University. Brewer's research interests include understanding the organizational culture, as well as healthcare professionals' and healthcare faculty members' EBP beliefs, and implementation that fosters best practices. Brewer teaches undergraduate, graduate, and DNP students evidence-based practice and serves on several doctoral committees. (Chapter 13)

Jacalyn S. Buck, PhD, RN, NEA-BC, is an Administrator for Nursing at The Ohio State University Wexner Medical Center. Buck has oversight for nursing quality, research, evidence-based practice, and nursing education across the health system. Her background is in maternal-child health and nursing administration, where she has served in a variety of roles ranging from Staff Nurse, Assistant Professor, and Director of Nursing to Nursing Administrator in various healthcare settings. She also serves as an Assistant Clinical Professor at The Ohio State University College of Nursing. Buck is a member of the American Nurses Association, American Organization of Nurse Executives, Ohio Hospital Association, Council on Graduate Education for Administration in Nursing, and Sigma Theta Tau International. (Chapter 11)

Sheila Chucta, MS, RN, CCRN, ACNS-BC, has been a registered nurse for 30 years. She received her bachelor of science in nursing from Capital University and her master's degree from The Ohio State University, where she also is pursuing her doctorate of nursing practice. Her career began at Rainbow Babies and Children's Hospital in the neonatal intensive-care unit; a year later she moved to The Ohio State University Medical Center and the adult patient population, where she continues to focus her energies. Her entire career has been focused on many aspects of critical care nursing, including medical, surgical, cardiac, transplant, and burn-patient populations. (Chapter 11)

Joanne Cleary-Holdforth, MSc, BSc, RGN, RM, has been a Lecturer in Nursing at Dublin City University since 2002. Her career began in Limerick, Ireland, where she trained as a general nurse and midwife at St. John's Hospital and the University Maternity Hospital, respectively. Cleary-Holdforth specialized in nephrology, dialysis, and transplantation at Beaumont Hospital, Dublin, the national referral center for renal transplantation. She completed her degree and master's in nursing at the Royal College of Surgeons in Ireland. Cleary-Holdforth is undertaking her PhD at Dublin City University, where she will explore the knowledge, understanding, and utilization of evidence-based practice (EBP) among nurses in Ireland. She completed the Evidence-Based Practice Mentorship Immersion Program at Arizona State University School of Nursing and Health Innovation in 2006 under the guidance of professors Bernadette Melnyk and Ellen Fineout-Overholt. (Chapter 5)

Deborah A. Francis, MS, BSN, RN-BC, ACNS-BC, has been a registered nurse for more than 25 years. She received her bachelor of science in nursing in 1988 and her master of science in 2010; she is completing her final semester of studies in the doctorate of nursing practice program from The Ohio State University College of Nursing. Francis is certified as a clinical nurse specialist and medical-surgical nurse. She is working as a clinical nurse specialist in the medical-surgical areas at The Ohio State University Wexner Medical Center. Francis has presented locally and nationally at the National Association of Clinical Nurse Specialists, Academy of Medical Surgical Nursing, and Ohio Organization of Nursing Executive conferences. (Chapter 11)

Julie Gerberick, MS, RN, CEN, is currently Education Nurse Specialist for Nationwide Children's Hospital in Columbus, Ohio, where she has spent her entire 25 years as a registered nurse. She is a master's prepared nurse in the field of child and adolescent health and has worked as an area specific educator for 16 years. (Chapter 12)

Tami Hartzell, MLS, is a Senior Librarian and nursing liaison at Rochester General Hospital, a 500-bed community hospital. She is a graduate of the first evidence-based practice (EBP) graduate certificate program in the country and and is an Expert EBP Mentor. In this role, Hartzell works closely with nursing staff to improve patient care by fostering a spirit of inquiry and coaching staff through the entire EBP process. Hartzell collaborates with the Evidence-Based Practice Advisory Council, Magnet® Steering Committee, and Nursing Research Council to develop and refine EBP processes and training for staff nurses. This collaboration has resulted in a three-time Magnet redesignation for Rochester General Hospital. (Chapter 4)

Pamela K. Lake, PhD, RN, AHN-BC, earned a bachelor of science in nursing from Texas Woman's University in 1975. After 25 years practicing in a variety of settings, she earned a master of science in nursing from the University of Texas at Tyler. She then taught for 16 years as a clinical instructor before she earned her PhD in 2013 from the University of Texas at Tyler, focusing on caring practice in nursing education. She is an Assistant Professor at the University of Texas at Tyler. Together with Ellen Fineout-Overholt, she reframed the undergraduate nursing research course into one focused on evidence-based decision-making and continues to work with faculty to diffuse evidence-based practice across the undergraduate curriculum. (Chapter 5)

Lisa English Long, MSN, RN, CNS, is an Instructor of Clinical Practice at The Ohio State University College of Nursing. Long received her bachelor of science in nursing from Eastern Kentucky University and master of science in nursing with a focus on parent-child health from the University of Cincinnati College of Nursing. Long furthered her education by attending Arizona State University College of Nursing and Health Innovation and completed the graduate certificate program in evidence-based practice (EBP). She is presently a doctoral candidate at the University of Louisville School of Nursing with a research focus on the state of the science of evidence-based practice, shared decision-making, and understanding healthcare professionals' and academic faculty's understanding of EBP and its impact on patient, family, staff, and organizational outcomes. Long teaches EBP and has led system changes toward a culture of EBP in academic and practice settings. (Chapter 13)

Tina L. Magers, PhD, RN-BC, is the Nursing Excellence and Research Coordinator at Mississippi Baptist Medical Center in Jackson, Mississippi. She received her PhD in nursing education and administration from William Carey University, her master of science in nursing from the University of Mississippi Medical Center, and her bachelor of science in nursing from Mississippi College. She is an Expert EBP Mentor and received a graduate certificate from Arizona State University School of Nursing and Health Innovation in evidence-based practice. She is board certified in nursing professional development. Magers' research and EBP interests include critical thinking of the new graduate, transition to practice, problem-based learning, and hospital-acquired infections. (Chapters 5 and 13)

Dónal O'Mathúna, PhD, received his bachelor of science in pharmacy from Trinity College in Dublin, Ireland, his PhD in medicinal chemistry from The Ohio State University, and his master of arts in theology/bioethics from Ashland University. He was Professor of Chemistry and Bioethics at Mount Carmel College of Nursing until 2002, when he returned to Ireland. There he is Senior Lecturer in Ethics, Decision-Making and Evidence in the School of Nursing & Human Sciences at Dublin City University. Since 2014, O'Mathúna has been Convenor of Cochrane Ireland, a role cofunded by the Ireland Health Research Board and Northern Ireland Research & Development Office to promote evidence-based practice (EBP) through the Cochrane Collaboration. O'Mathúna has been actively involved in the Cochrane Collaboration since 1998, is a co-author of five published Cochrane systematic reviews, and is supervising four ongoing Cochrane reviews. He coordinates training in systematic reviews across the island of Ireland, presents internationally on EBP, and has peer-reviewed publications in journals and textbooks. (Chapter 5)

Brenda K. Vermillion, DNP, RN, CCRN, ACNS-BC, ANP-BC, has been a registered nurse for 30 years. She received her bachelor of science in nursing, her master of science in nursing, and her doctor of nursing practice from The Ohio State University. She holds certifications as a clinical nurse specialist and an adult nurse practitioner. In 2013, she was appointed as Director of Health System Nursing Education at The Ohio State University Wexner Medical Center and Assistant Clinical Professor for The Ohio State University College of Nursing (OSUCON). Vermillion is an evidence-based practice mentor, teaches evidence-based nursing scholarship for the master's prepared nurse at The OSUCON, and has authored and co-authored numerous evidence-based practice guidelines for her organization. Vermillion has been a presenter at multiple conferences related to critical care nursing and continues to be involved with the American Association of Critical-Care Nurses, Society of Critical Care Medicine, Association of Nursing Professional Development, and American Organization of Nurse Executives. (Chapter 11)

Michele L. Weber, DNP, RN, CCRN, OCN, CCNS, APN-BC, received her bachelor of science in nursing from DePauw University and her master of science in nursing and doctor of nursing practice degrees from The Ohio State University. Weber holds active certificates of authority as a clinical nurse specialist and an adult nurse practitioner. For the past 10 years, she has worked as a clinical nurse specialist throughout all the intensive care units. She holds an active appointment as a Clinical Assistant Professor through The Ohio State University College of Nursing. Weber is an expert in clinical care of complex and critically ill patients as well as an expert in the translation of evidence-based practice into bedside clinical practice. She has presented at numerous local, regional, national, and international conferences on a variety of nursing topics. (Chapter 11)

TABLE OF CONTENTS

About the Authors viii
Contributing Authors xiii
Introduction xxii

I   INTRODUCTION TO THE EVIDENCE-BASED
     PRACTICE COMPETENCIES 1

1   THE FOUNDATION FOR IMPROVING HEALTHCARE QUALITY,
     PATIENT OUTCOMES, & COSTS WITH EVIDENCE-BASED
     PRACTICE 3
        Setting the Stage 4
        Evidence-based Practice and the Quadruple Aim in Healthcare 5
        Definition of Evidence-based Practice 8
        The Seven Steps of Evidence-based Practice 10
        Rationale for the New EBP Competencies 16
        Summary 16
        References 16

2   DEVELOPMENT OF AND EVIDENCE TO SUPPORT THE
     EVIDENCE-BASED PRACTICE COMPETENCIES 19
        Setting the Stage 20
        Importance of Evidence-based Practice Competencies 21
        Implications for Use of the EBP Competencies 28
        Summary 29
        References 29

II   ACHIEVING COMPETENCY WITH THE EVIDENCE-
     BASED PRACTICE COMPETENCIES 31

3   THE EVIDENCE-BASED PRACTICE COMPETENCIES RELATED
     TO CLINICAL INQUIRY 33
        Setting the Stage 34
        Clinical Inquiry Defined and Described 35
        Building a Culture That Supports Clinical Inquiry 36
        Summary 53
        References 54

4   THE EVIDENCE-BASED PRACTICE COMPETENCIES
    RELATED TO SEARCHING FOR BEST EVIDENCE 55
        Setting the Stage 56
        Developing a Systematic Approach to Searching 58
        Summary 74
        References 74

5   THE EVIDENCE-BASED PRACTICE COMPETENCIES
    RELATED TO CRITICAL APPRAISAL: RAPID CRITICAL
    APPRAISAL, EVALUATION, SYNTHESIS, AND
    RECOMMENDATIONS 77
        Setting the Stage 78
        Understanding the Critical Appraisal Process. 81
        Taking a Group Approach to Critical Appraisal 89
        Summary. 106
        References 106

6   THE EVIDENCE-BASED PRACTICE COMPETENCIES
    RELATED TO IMPLEMENTATION 109
        Setting the Stage 110
        Implementing an Evidence-based Practice Change:
            Planning for Change. 112
        Tools to Guide the EBP Change Process 114
        Summary. 128
        References 128

7   THE EVIDENCE-BASED PRACTICE COMPETENCIES
    RELATED TO OUTCOMES EVALUATION 129
        Setting the Stage 130
        Evaluating Outcomes 131
        Summary. 141
        References 141

8   THE EVIDENCE-BASED PRACTICE COMPETENCIES
    RELATED TO LEADING AND SUSTAINING EVIDENCE-
    BASED PRACTICE 143
        Setting the Stage 144
        Essential Components of an Evidence-based Practice Culture and
            Environment. 145

The ARCC Model: A System-Wide Framework for Implementing and
    Sustaining EBP 151
Summary 159
References 160

9   **THE EVIDENCE-BASED PRACTICE COMPETENCIES
RELATED TO DISSEMINATING EVIDENCE** **163**
Setting the Stage 164
The Importance of Disseminating Evidence 164
Summary 181
References 181

III **A PRACTICAL GUIDE TO INTEGRATING THE
EVIDENCE-BASED PRACTICE COMPETENCIES
IN DIFFERENT ROLES.** **183**

10 **INTEGRATING THE EVIDENCE-BASED PRACTICE
COMPETENCIES IN HEALTHCARE SETTINGS** **185**
Strategies for Integrating the EBP Competencies in Healthcare
    Settings 186
Calculating the ROI of EBP 195
Developing Educational Programs around EBP Competencies 198
Creating Opportunities for Interprofessional Learning and
    Collaboration 201
Developing Other Skills 201
Examples of Integration of the EBP Competencies 202
Summary 202
References 203

11 **INTEGRATING THE EVIDENCE-BASED PRACTICE
COMPETENCIES INTO THE ROLE OF ADVANCED
PRACTICE NURSES** **205**
Clinical Nurse Specialists' Role in EBP 207
The CNS as an EBP Mentor 209
The CNS and the EBP Competencies. 210
Building the Infrastructure for EBP at an Academic Medical Center
    Through the Role of the CNS 211
Summary 222
References 222

12 USING THE EVIDENCE-BASED PRACTICE COMPETENCIES
    WITH POLICY AND PROCEDURE COMMITTEES 225
        EBP Competency and the Patient/Family Care Policy Committee......... 226
        A Cost-Effective EBP Competency Assessment and Education........... 228
        Determining an Interprofessional Education Framework 229
        Challenges to Using the Evidence-based Practice Competencies
          with Policy and Procedure Committees............................. 234
        Development of a Unit-Based EBP Policy: A Personal Narrative 237
        Summary.. 243
        References 244

13 TEACHING THE EVIDENCE-BASED PRACTICE
    COMPETENCIES IN CLINICAL AND ACADEMIC SETTINGS ... 245
        Matching EBP Competencies to Existing Standards 249
        Teaching and Evaluation Strategies for Incorporating EBP
          Competencies 262
        Summary.. 273
        References 273

IV APPENDIXES 277

 A PICOT WORKSHEET AND SEARCH STRATEGY
    DEVELOPMENT 279

 B EXAMPLE OF A COMPLETED GENERAL APPRAISAL
    OVERVIEW (GAO) 283

 C EXAMPLE OF A COMPLETED RAPID CRITICAL APPRAISAL
    CHECKLIST WITH RATIONALE 287

 D EVALUATION TABLE TEMPLATE........................... 293

    GLOSSARY 297

    INDEX... 309

INTRODUCTION

Knowing is not enough; we must apply.
Willing is not enough; we must do.
–Goethe

This famous quote by Goethe is so pertinent to evidence-based practice (EBP) given that we have an enormous body of published knowledge from research available, yet so little of it is implemented in healthcare settings. It continues to take years, often decades, to translate findings from research into clinical practice to improve healthcare quality and outcomes. Unfortunately, for much of our scientific body of published research, it is never used.

We have long described the barriers and facilitators to EBP, but healthcare systems and clinicians still face many barriers and "character-builders" in implementing and sustaining evidence-based care. Some of these barriers are decades old, but a new barrier that we recently identified through a national survey with nurses across the country is resistance to EBP by nurse leaders and managers. This barrier is significant because if nurse leaders and managers do not "walk the talk" of EBP and create cultures and environments that support clinicians to implement evidence-based care, it will not happen or sustain. The data from this national nursing survey and the findings from a more recent survey with chief nursing executives and chief nursing officers that revealed low prioritization of EBP and little budgetary investment in it prompted us to conduct a national summit with more than 150 chief nurse leaders. The purpose of this summit was to share the data from these two national studies and obtain the chief nurse leaders' feedback regarding resources, educational offerings, and tools that could assist them in creating EBP cultures and environments that sustain. The leaders attending the summit said that they needed more knowledge and skills in EBP themselves along with tools to help them support and advance EBP in their institutions. For many years, we also have heard the same request from clinicians for more tools that would help them to implement and sustain EBP. Therefore, we have responded to these requests by developing this book, which provides a practical tool kit for implementing the new EBP competencies in real-world practice settings.

For years, clinicians, leaders, and faculty have struggled with what it means to be competent in EBP. However, there were no research-based EBP competencies for practicing registered nurses (RNs) and advanced practice nurses (APNs) that could set the standard for evidence-based decision-making and care and eliminate the confusion regarding what exactly competency in EBP means. Therefore, we embarked on a journey to develop research-based EBP competencies that could serve as a guide for establishing and assessing EBP competence in RNs and APNs.

In this book, you will read about the vital importance of EBP and learn how the EBP competencies were developed. In addition, this book provides markers of competence for each EBP competency as well as assessment strategies that facilitate implementation of the competencies in real-world clinical settings. The primary goals of this book are to serve as a practical guide for clinicians, leaders, faculty, EBP mentors, and students that will assist them in achieving competency in EBP, facilitate evidence-based decision-making in daily practice, and help sustain evidence-based care as part of a mission to create an EBP enterprise that can accelerate the speed at which research knowledge is translated into real-world settings to improve health outcomes and decrease healthcare costs. Each chapter begins and ends with case scenarios that illustrate exemplars of how the competencies can be actively implemented and assessed in clinical settings.

Numerous hospitals and healthcare systems across the nation and world are trying to build and sustain EBP cultures and environments, yet they struggle with how exactly to accomplish that goal as well as how to know when their institution has "arrived" in EBP. Some institutions believe they have arrived when they have two or three EBP projects underway. Other institutions say they have arrived or excel in evidence-based care when they have purchased an electronic EBP resource. Although these are steps in an EBP journey, an institution has not arrived until EBP is in the DNA of the entire organization and every person who works within it, and also when evidence-based decision-making and evidence-based care are consistently the norm. This book is intended to provide practical advice and ready-to-use resources to help organizations integrate EBP broadly across and deeply into their infrastructure. A widely dispersed and multicomponent strategy is far more likely to move an organization from one that dabbles in

EBP occasionally to an organization that is hard-wired for EBP. We have made it standard practice to always ask the following two questions routinely when we are working with clinicians, leaders, faculty, and students:

What will you do in the next 3 to 5 years if you know that you cannot fail?

What is the smallest EBP change that you can make TODAY that will improve the health of the people for whom you care?

We must remember that "nothing happens unless first we dream" (Carl Sandburg). We must dream something before we can do it. Yet in today's world, so many people lose their dreams because of well-meaning people who talk about all the reasons why something cannot happen instead of how it can happen. We ask everyone we work with to write down their dreams and goals, put a date on them, and place them in an area that is seen every morning and every night. Research has shown that when we write down our dreams and goals and view them every day, we will move faster in accomplishing them. However, the keys to accomplishing dreams are belief in one's ability to accomplish them and persistent action to make them happen. Therefore, the time to act with a sense of urgency is *now*! We have so much knowledge available to improve the quality of healthcare and health outcomes, yet we so often do not use it. We must always remember that although changing the way we approach practice is a steep climb, it is a climb that we are obligated as professionals to make. Our patients, families, and communities are depending on us. They expect us to be current and evidence-based in our practice. That is what any of us would hope for and expect from a healthcare team caring for one of our loved ones. This is the dream and the challenge. We hope this book will serve as your guide and assist you in meeting this challenge and seeing your dream for EBP come to fruition.

–*Bernadette Mazurek Melnyk, Lynn Gallagher-Ford, and Ellen Fineout-Overholt*

INTRODUCTION TO THE EVIDENCE-BASED PRACTICE COMPETENCIES

In Chapters 1 and 2, you'll learn about the vital importance of EBP and how the EBP competencies were developed.

Chapter 1. 3

Chapter 2. 19

THE FOUNDATION FOR IMPROVING HEALTHCARE QUALITY, PATIENT OUTCOMES, & COSTS WITH EVIDENCE-BASED PRACTICE

Bernadette Mazurek Melnyk, PhD, RN, CPNP/PMHNP, FAANP, FNAP, FAAN

KEY CONTENT IN THIS CHAPTER

- Evidence-based practice and the Quadruple Aim in healthcare

- Definition of evidence-based practice

- The Seven Steps of evidence-based practice

- Rationale for the evidence-based practice competencies

To know and not to do is really not to know.

–Stephen R. Covey

SETTING THE STAGE

Have you ever wondered why the United States spends more money on healthcare than any western country, yet it ranks 37th in world health outcomes? Have you ever questioned why patients are awakened every 2 to 4 hours for vital signs in the hospital when they are stable and in desperate need of sleep? Or wondered why nurses work 12-hour shifts when research shows the multiple adverse outcomes of working lengthy hours for both clinicians and patients? Have you ever thought about the millions of healthcare dollars that could be saved if all primary care providers would follow the evidence-based recommendations of the U.S. Preventive Services Task Force? Have you ever questioned why it often takes decades for the evidence that is generated from research to be translated into the real world to improve healthcare quality and patient outcomes?

Tina Magers (nursing professional development and research coordinator at Mississippi Baptist Health Systems) and her team wondered why catheter-associated urinary tract infections (CAUTIs) affect as many as 25% of all hospitalized patients and questioned what evidence exists that could inform a practice change to reduce these infections in their hospital. (This is Step #0 in the seven-step evidence-based practice [EBP] process, which we describe in detail later in this chapter.) As a result, the team formed the following question in a format called PICOT (Patient population, Intervention or Interest area, Comparison intervention or group, Outcome, and Time; Step #1 in EBP) that facilitated them to conduct an expedited effective search for the best evidence (Magers, 2015):

In adult patients hospitalized in a long-term acute care hospital (P), how does the use of a nurse-driven protocol for evaluating the appropriateness of short-term urinary catheter continuation or removal (I) compared to no protocol (C) affect the number of catheter days and CAUTI rates (O) over a six-month post-intervention period (T)?

The team conducted an evidence search to answer this clinical question using the Cumulative Index to Nursing and Allied Health Literature (CINAHL), the Cochrane Database of Systematic Reviews, Cochrane Central Register of

Controlled Trials, the Database of Abstracts of Reviews of Effects (DARE), Ovid Clinical Queries, and PubMed (Step #2 in EBP), followed by rapid critical appraisal of 15 studies found in the search (Step #3 in EBP). A synthesis of the 15 studies led the team to conclude that early removal of urinary catheters would likely reduce catheter days and CAUTIs (the identified outcomes). Therefore, the team wrote a protocol based on the evidence, listing eight criteria for the continuation of a short-term urinary catheter (Step #4 in EBP).

After the protocol was presented to the medical executive committee at their hospital for approval, a process for the change was put into practice, including an education plan with an algorithm that was implemented in small group inservices for the nurses, posters, and written handouts for physicians. An outcomes evaluation (Step #5 in the EBP process) revealed a significant reduction in catheter days and a clinically significant reduction of 33% in CAUTIs. The team disseminated the outcomes of the project to internal audiences (e.g., their Nursing Quality Council, the EBP and Research Council, Nursing Leadership Council, Organization Infection Control Committee) and external venues (presentations at regional conferences and a publication in the *American Journal of Nursing*) (Magers, 2013). (Step #6 in the EBP process.)

This is a stellar exemplar of how a team with a spirit of inquiry and a commitment to improving healthcare quality can use the seven-step EBP process discussed in this chapter to improve patient outcomes and reduce hospital costs.

EVIDENCE-BASED PRACTICE AND THE QUADRUPLE AIM IN HEALTHCARE

Findings from an extensive body of research support that EBP improves the quality and safety of healthcare, enhances health outcomes, decreases geographic variation in care, and reduces costs (McGinty & Anderson, 2008; Melnyk & Fineout-Overholt, 2015; Melnyk, Fineout-Overholt, Gallagher-Ford, & Kaplan,

2012a). In the United States, EBP has been recognized as a key factor in meeting the Triple Aim in healthcare, defined as (Berwick, Nolan, & Whittington, 2008):

- Improving the patient experience of care (including quality and satisfaction)

- Improving the health of populations

- Reducing the per capita cost of healthcare

The Triple Aim has now been expanded to the Quadruple Aim: the fourth goal being to improve work life and decrease burnout in clinicians (Bodenheimer & Sinsky, 2014).

Because EBP has been found to empower clinicians and result in higher levels of job satisfaction (Strout, 2005), it also can assist healthcare systems in achieving the Quadruple Aim. However, regardless of its tremendous positive outcomes, EBP is not standard of care in healthcare systems throughout the United States or the rest of the world due to multiple barriers that have continued to persist over the past decades. Some of these barriers include (Melnyk & Fineout-Overholt, 2015; Melnyk et al., 2012a; Melnyk et al., 2012b; Melnyk et al., 2016; Pravikoff, Pierce, & Tanner, 2005; Titler, 2009):

- Inadequate knowledge and skills in EBP by nurses and other healthcare professionals

- Lack of cultures and environments that support EBP

- Misperceptions that EBP takes too much time

- Outdated organizational politics and policies

- Limited resources and tools available for point-of-care providers, including budgetary investment in EBP by chief nurse executives

- Resistance from colleagues, nurse managers, and leaders

- Inadequate numbers of EBP mentors in healthcare systems

- Academic programs that continue to teach baccalaureat, master's, and doctor of nursing practice students the rigorous process of how to conduct research instead of taking an evidence-based approach to care

Urgent action is needed to rapidly accelerate EBP in order to reduce the tremendously long lag between the generation of research findings and their implementation in clinical settings. Many interventions or treatments that have been found to improve outcomes through research are not standard of care throughout healthcare systems or have never been used in clinical settings. It took more than 20 years for neonatal and pediatric intensive care units to adopt the Creating Opportunities for Parent Empowerment (COPE) Program for parents of preterm infants and critically ill children even though multiple intervention studies supported that COPE reduced parent depression and anxiety, enhanced parental-infant interaction, and improved child outcomes (Melnyk & Fineout-Overholt, 2015). It was not until findings from a National Institute of Nursing Research funded randomized controlled trial supported that COPE reduced neonatal intensive care unit (NICU) length of stay in premature infants by 4 days (8 days in preterms less than 32 weeks) and its associated substantial decreased costs that NICUs across the country began to implement the intervention as standard of care (Melnyk & Feinstein, 2009; Melnyk et al., 2006).

If not for an improvement in "so-what" outcomes (outcomes of importance to the healthcare system, such as decreased length of stay and costs), COPE would not have been translated into NICU settings to improve outcomes in vulnerable children and their families. On the other hand, many interventions or practices that do not have a solid body of evidence to support them continue to be implemented in healthcare, including double-checking pediatric medications, assessing nasogastric tube placement with air, and taking vital signs every 2 or 4 hours for hospitalized patients. These practices that are steeped in tradition instead of based upon the best evidence result in less than optimum care, poor outcomes, and wasteful healthcare spending.

DEFINITION OF EVIDENCE-BASED PRACTICE

As EBP evolved, it was defined as the conscientious use of current best evidence to make decisions about patient care (Sackett, Straus, Richardson, Rosenberg, & Haynes, 2000). Since this earlier definition, EBP has been broadened to include a lifelong problem-solving approach to how healthcare is delivered that integrates the best evidence from high-quality studies with a clinician's expertise and also a patient's preferences and values (Melnyk & Fineout-Overholt, 2015; see Figure 1.1). Incorporated within a clinician's expertise are:

- Clinical judgment

- Internal evidence from the patient's history and physical exam, as well as data gathered from EBP, quality improvement, or outcomes management projects

- An evaluation of available resources required to deliver the best practices

Some barriers inhibit the uptake of EBP across all venues and disciplines within healthcare. Although the strongest level of evidence that guides clinical practice interventions (i.e., Level I evidence) are systematic reviews of randomized controlled trials followed by well-designed randomized controlled trials (i.e., Level II evidence), there is a limited number of systematic reviews and intervention studies in the nursing profession. Single descriptive quantitative and qualitative studies, which are considered lower-level evidence, continue to dominate the field; see Table 1.1 for levels of evidence that are used to guide clinical interventions.

However, all studies that are relevant to the clinical question should be included in the body of evidence that guides clinical practice. In addition, clinicians often lack critical appraisal skills needed to determine the quality of evidence that is produced by research. Critical appraisal of evidence is an essential step in EBP given that strength or level of evidence plus quality of that evidence gives clinicians the confidence to act and change practice. If Level I evidence is published but is found to lack rigor and be of poor quality through critical appraisal, a clinician would not want to make a practice change based on that evidence.

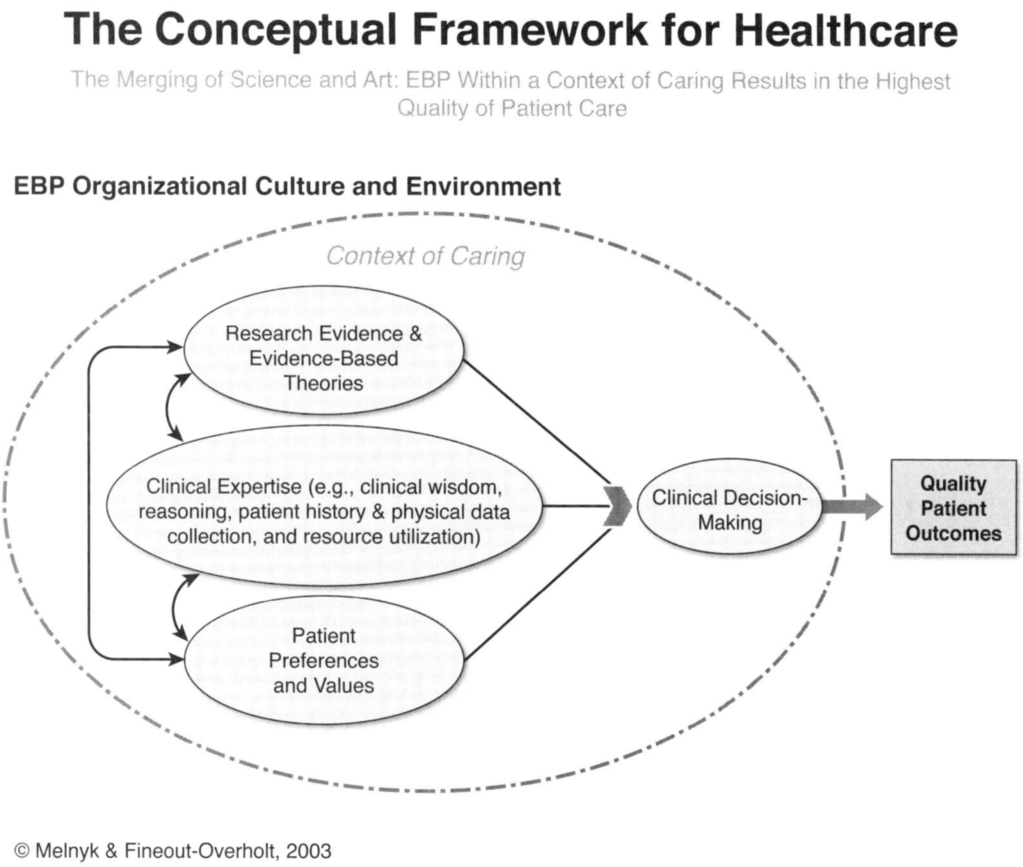

The Conceptual Framework for Healthcare

The Merging of Science and Art: EBP Within a Context of Caring Results in the Highest Quality of Patient Care

EBP Organizational Culture and Environment

© Melnyk & Fineout-Overholt, 2003

Figure 1.1   Components of an EBP within a culture and environment that support it lead to the best clinical decisions and patient outcomes.

TABLE 1.1 RATING SYSTEM FOR THE HIERARCHY OF EVIDENCE TO GUIDE CLINICAL INTERVENTIONS

Level	Explanation
I	Evidence from a systematic review or meta-analysis of all relevant randomized controlled trials (RCTs)
II	Evidence obtained from well-designed RCTs
III	Evidence obtained from well-designed controlled trials without randomization
IV	Evidence from well-designed case-control and cohort studies
V	Evidence from systematic reviews of descriptive and qualitative studies
VI	Evidence from single descriptive or qualitative studies
VII	Evidence from the opinion of authorities and/or reports of expert committees

Source: Modified from Elwyn et al. (2015) and Harris et al. (2001).

THE SEVEN STEPS OF EVIDENCE-BASED PRACTICE

Evidence-based practice was originally described as a five-step process including (Sackett et al., 2000):

1. Ask the clinical question in PICOT format.

2. Search for the best evidence.

3. Critically appraise the evidence.

4. Integrate the evidence with a clinician's expertise and a patient's preferences and values.

5. Evaluate the outcome of the practice change.

In 2011, Melnyk and Fineout-Overholt added two additional steps to the process, resulting in the following seven-step EBP process (see Table 1.2).

TABLE 1.2 THE SEVEN STEPS OF EVIDENCE-BASED PRACTICE

Step	Explanation
0	Cultivate a spirit of inquiry within an EBP culture and environment.
1	Ask the burning clinical question in PICOT format.
2	Search for and collect the most relevant best evidence.
3	Critically appraise the evidence (i.e., rapid critical appraisal, evaluation, synthesis, and recommendations).
4	Integrate the best evidence with one's clinical expertise and patient preferences and values in making a practice decision or change.
5	Evaluate outcomes of the practice decision or change based on evidence.
6	Disseminate the outcomes of the EBP decision or change.

Step #0: Cultivate a Spirit of Inquiry Within an EBP Culture and Environment

The first step in EBP is to cultivate a spirit of inquiry, which is a continual questioning of clinical practices. When delivering care to patients, it is important to consistently question current practices: For example, is Prozac or Zoloft more effective in treating adolescents with depression? Does use of bronchodilators with metered dose inhalers (MDIs) and spacers versus nebulizers in the emergency department (ED) with asthmatic children lead to better oxygenation levels? Does double-checking pediatric medications lead to fewer medication errors?

Cultures and environments that support a spirit of inquiry are more likely to facilitate and sustain a questioning spirit in clinicians. Some key components of an EBP culture and environment include (Melnyk, 2014; Melnyk & Fineout-Overholt, 2015; Melnyk et al., 2012a, 2016):

- An organizational vision, mission, and goals that include EBP

- An infrastructure with EBP tools and resources

- Orientation sessions for new clinicians that communicate an expectation of delivering evidence-based care and meeting the EBP competencies for practicing registered nurses (RNs) and advanced practice nurses (APNs)

- Leaders and managers who "walk the talk" and support their clinicians to deliver evidence-based care

- A critical mass of EBP mentors to work with point-of-care clinicians in facilitating evidence-based care

- Evidence-based policies and procedures

- Orientations and ongoing professional development seminars that provide EBP knowledge and skills-building along with an expectation for EBP

- Integration of the EBP competencies in performance evaluations and clinical ladders

- Recognition programs that reward evidence-based care

Step #1: Ask the Burning Clinical Question in PICOT Format

After a clinician asks a clinical question, it is important to place that question in PICOT format to facilitate an evidence search that is effective in getting to the best evidence in an efficient manner. PICOT represents:

- P: Patient population

- I: Intervention or Interest area

- C: Comparison intervention or group

- O: Outcome

- T: Time (if relevant)

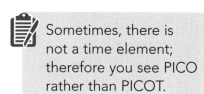

Sometimes, there is not a time element; therefore you see PICO rather than PICOT.

For example, the clinical questions asked in Step #0 that all involve interventions or treatments should be rephrased in the following PICOT format to result in the most efficient and effective database searches:

- In depressed adolescents (P), how does Prozac (I) compared to Zoloft (C) affect depressive symptoms (O) 3 months after starting treatment (T)?

- In asthmatic children seen in the ED (P), how do bronchodilators delivered with MDIs with spacers (I) compared to nebulizers (C) affect oxygenation levels (O) 1 hour after treatment (T)?

- In hospitalized children (P), how does double-checking pediatric medications with a second nurse (I) compared to not double-checking (C) affect medication errors (O) during a 30-day time period (T)?

In addition to intervention or treatment questions, other types of PICOT questions include meaning questions, diagnosis questions, etiology questions, and prognosis questions that are addressed in Chapter 3.

Step #2: Search for and Collect the Most Relevant Best Evidence

After the clinical question is placed in PICOT format with the proper template, each keyword in the PICOT question should be used to systematically search for the best evidence; this strategy is referred to as *keyword searching*. For example, to gather the evidence to answer the intervention PICOT questions in Step #1, you would first search databases for systematic reviews and randomized controlled trials given that they are the strongest levels of evidence to guide practice decisions.

 A few databases you'll want to get familiar with are Cochrane Database of Systematic Reviews, MEDLINE, and CINAHL.

However, the search should extend to include all evidence that answers the clinical question. Each keyword or phrase from the PICOT question (e.g., depressed adolescents, Prozac, Zoloft, depressive symptoms) should be entered individually and searched. Searching controlled vocabulary that matches the keywords is the next step in a systematic approach to searching.

In the final step, combine each keyword and controlled vocabulary previously searched, which typically yields a small number of studies that should answer the PICOT question. This systematic approach to searching for evidence typically yields a small number of studies to answer the clinical question versus a less systematic approach, which usually produces a large number of irrelevant studies. More specific information about searching is covered in Chapter 4.

Step #3: Critically Appraise the Evidence

After relevant evidence has been found, critical appraisal begins. First, it is important to conduct a rapid critical appraisal (RCA) of each study from the data search to determine whether they are *keeper studies*: that is, they indeed answer the clinical question. This process includes answering the following questions:

- **Are the results of the study valid?** Did the researchers use the best methods to conduct the study (study validity)? For example, assessment of a study's validity determines whether the methods used to conduct the study were rigorous.

- **What are the results?** Do the results matter, and can I get similar results in my practice (study reliability)?

- **Will the results help me in caring for my patients?** Is the treatment feasible to use with my patients (study applicability)?

Rapid critical appraisal checklists can assist clinicians in evaluating validity, reliability, and applicability of a study in a time-efficient way. See Chapter 5 for one example of an RCA checklist for randomized controlled trials and Melnyk & Fineout-Overholt (2015) for a variety of RCA checklists. After an RCA is completed on each study and found to be a keeper, it is included in the evaluation and synthesis of the body evidence to determine whether a practice change should be made. Chapter 5 contains more information on critically appraising, evaluating, and synthesizing evidence.

Step #4: Integrate the Best Evidence with One's Clinical Expertise and Patient Preferences and Values in Making a Practice Decision or Change

After the body of evidence from the search is critically appraised, evaluated, and synthesized, it should be integrated with a clinician's expertise and also a patient's preferences and values to determine whether the practice change should be conducted. Providing the patient with evidence-based information and involving him or her in the decision regarding whether he or she should receive a certain intervention is an important step in EBP. To facilitate greater involvement of patients in making decisions about their care in collaboration with healthcare providers, there has been an accelerated movement in creating and testing patient-decision support tools, which provide evidence-based information in a relatable understandable format (Elwyn et al., 2015).

Step #5: Evaluate Outcomes of the Practice Decision or Change Based on Evidence

After making a practice change based on the best evidence, it is critical to evaluate outcomes—the consequences of an intervention or treatment. For example, an outcome of providing a baby with a pacifier might be a decrease in crying. Outcomes evaluation is essential to determine the impact of the practice changes on healthcare quality and health outcomes. It is important to target "so-what" outcomes that the current healthcare system considers important, such as complication rates, length of stay, rehospitalization rates, and costs given that hospitals are currently being reimbursed based on their performance on these outcomes (Melnyk & Morrison-Beedy, 2012). A more thorough discussion of approaches to outcomes evaluation is included in Chapter 7.

Step #6: Disseminate the Outcomes of the EBP Decision or Change

Silos often exist, even within the same healthcare organization. So that others can benefit from the positive changes resulting from EBP, it is important to disseminate the findings. Various avenues for dissemination include institutional EBP rounds; poster and podium presentations at local, regional, and national conferences; and publications. More detailed information about disseminating outcomes of EBP is included in Chapter 9.

RATIONALE FOR THE NEW EBP COMPETENCIES

To accelerate the uptake of EBP and ensure that nurses are competent in the delivery of evidence-based care, a new set of EBP competencies was recently developed for practicing RNs and APNs. Competencies are typically developed and used to ensure the delivery of high-quality, safe nursing care, which should be an expectation from the public (American Nurses Association, 2010; Melnyk, Gallagher-Ford, Long, & Fineout-Overholt, 2014). The process of developing these competencies along with the research conducted to further validate them are described in Chapter 2.

SUMMARY

This chapter discussed how evidence-based practice (EBP) improves healthcare quality, patient outcomes, and cost reductions, yet multiple barriers persist in healthcare settings that need to be rapidly overcome. Ensuring that clinicians meet the newly established EBP competencies along with creating cultures and environments that support EBP are key strategies to transform the current state of nursing practice and healthcare delivery to its highest level.

REFERENCES

American Nurses Association. (2010). *Nursing: Scope and standards of practice* (2nd edition). Silver Spring, MD: American Nurses Association.

Berwick, D. M., Nolan, T. W., & Whittington, J. (2008). The Triple Aim: Care, health, and cost. *Health Affairs, 27*(3), 759–769.

Bodenheimer, T., & Sinsky, C. (2014). From Triple to Quadruple Aim: Care of the patient requires care of the provider. *Annals of Family Medicine, 12,* 573–576.

Elwyn, G., Quinlan, C., Mulley, A., Agoritsas, T., Vandik, P. O., & Guyatt, G. (2015). Trustworthy guidelines—excellent; customized care tools—even better. *BioMed Central Medicine, 13*(1), 199. Modified from Guyatt, G., & Rennie, D. (2002), *Users' guides to the medical literature.* Chicago, IL: American Medical Association.

Harris, R. P., Hefland, M., Woolf, S. H., Lohr, K. N., Mulrow, C. D., Teutsch, S. M., & Atkins, D. (2001). Current methods of the U.S. Preventive Services Task Force: A review of the process. *American Journal of Preventive Medicine, 20,* 21–35.

Magers, T. (2013). Using evidence-based practice to reduce catheter-associated urinary tract infections. *American Journal of Nursing, 113*(6), 34–42.

Magers, T. L. (2015). Using evidence-based practice to reduce catheter-associated urinary tract infections in a long-term acute care facility. In B. M. Melnyk & E. Fineout-Overholt (Eds.), *Evidence-based practice in nursing & healthcare. A guide to best practice* (3rd ed.) (pp. 70–73). Philadelphia, PA: Wolters Kluwer.

McGinty, J., & Anderson, G. (2008). Predictors of physician compliance with American Heart Association guidelines for acute myocardial infarction. *Critical Care Nursing Quarterly, 31*(2), 161–172.

Melnyk, B. M. (2014). Building cultures and environments that facilitate clinician behavior change to evidence-based practice: What works? *Worldviews on Evidence-Based Nursing, 11*(2), 79–80.

Melnyk, B. M., & Fineout-Overholt, E. (2011). *Evidence-based practice in nursing & healthcare. A guide to best practice* (pp. 1–24). Philadelphia, PA: Wolters Kluwer/Lippincott Williams & Wilkins.

Melnyk, B. M., & Fineout-Overholt, E. (2015). *Evidence-based practice in nursing & healthcare. A guide to best practice* (3rd ed.) (pp. 3–23). Philadelphia, PA: Wolters Kluwer.

Melnyk, B. M., Fineout-Overholt, E., Gallagher-Ford, L., & Kaplan, L. (2012a). The state of evidence-based practice in US nurses: Critical implications for nurse leaders and educators. *Journal of Nursing Administration, 42*(9), 410–417.

Melnyk, B. M., Grossman, D., Chou, R., Mabry-Hernandez, I., Nicholson, W., Dewitt, T.G. . . . & Flores, G. (2012b). USPSTF perspective on evidence-based preventive recommendations for children. *Pediatrics, 130*(2), e399–e407.

Melnyk, B. M., & Feinstein, N. (2009). Reducing hospital expenditures with the COPE (Creating Opportunities for Parent Empowerment) program for parents and premature infants: An analysis of direct healthcare neonatal intensive care unit costs and savings. *Nursing Administrative Quarterly, 33*(1), 32–37.

Melnyk, B. M., Feinstein, N. F., Alpert-Gillis, L., Fairbanks, E., Crean, H. F., Sinkin, R., & Gross, S. J. (2006). Reducing premature infants' length of stay and improving parents' mental health outcomes with the COPE NICU program: A randomized clinical trial. *Pediatrics, 118*(5), e1414–e1427.

Melnyk, B. M., Gallagher-Ford, L., Thomas, B. K., Troseth, M., Wyngarden, K., & Szalacha, L. (2016). A study of chief nurse executives indicates low prioritization of evidence-based practice and shortcomings in hospital performance metrics across the United States. *Worldviews on Evidence-Based Nursing, 13*(1), 6–14.

Melnyk, B. M., Gallagher-Ford, L., Long, L., & Fineout-Overholt, E. (2014). The establishment of evidence-based practice competencies for practicing nurses and advanced practice nurses in real-world clinical settings: Proficiencies to improve healthcare quality, reliability, patient outcomes, and costs. *Worldviews on Evidence-Based Nursing, 11*(1), 5–15.

Melnyk, B. M., & Morrison-Beedy, D. (2012). Setting the stage for intervention research: The "so what," "what exists" and "what's next" factors. In B. M. Melnyk & D. Morrison-Beedy (Eds.), *Designing, conducting, analyzing and funding intervention research. A practical guide for success* (pp. 1–9). New York, NY: Springer Publishing Company.

Pravikoff, D. S., Pierce, S. T., & Tanner A. (2005). Evidence-based practice readiness study supported by academy nursing informatics expert panel. *Nursing Outlook, 53*(1), 49–50.

Sackett, D. L., Straus, S. E., Richardson, W. S., Rosenberg, W., & Haynes, R. B. (2000). *Evidence-based medicine: How to practice and teach EBM.* London, UK: Churchill Livingstone.

Strout, T. D. (2005). Curiosity and reflective thinking: Renewal of the spirit. In Clinical scholars at the bedside: An EBP mentorship model for today [electronic version]. *Excellence in Nursing Knowledge.* Indianapolis, IN: Sigma Theta Tau International.

Titler, M. G. (2009). Developing an evidence-based practice. In G. LoBiondo-Wood & J. Haber (Eds.), *Nursing research: Methods and critical appraisal for evidence-based practice* (7th ed.) (pp. 385–437). St Louis, MO: Mosby.

2

DEVELOPMENT OF AND EVIDENCE TO SUPPORT THE EVIDENCE-BASED PRACTICE COMPETENCIES

Bernadette Mazurek Melnyk, PhD, RN, CPNP/PMHNP, FAANP, FNAP, FAAN

KEY CONTENT IN THIS CHAPTER

- Importance of evidence-based practice (EBP) competencies

- Phase I development and validation of the EBP competencies

- Phase II validation of the EBP competencies through research

- Implications for use of the EBP competencies

> If you are going to achieve excellence in big things, you develop the habit in little matters. Excellence is not an exception, it is a prevailing attitude.
>
> —Colin Powell

SETTING THE STAGE

Trish is a newly appointed master's-prepared nurse manager of a 22-bed surgical intensive care unit (ICU) housed within a large urban academic medical center. Her goal is to be the lead unit in the hospital for evidence-based practice (EBP) with the highest quality of care and best patient outcomes, including zero rates of ventilator-associated pneumonia, pressure ulcers, and secondary infections. The unit has experienced much nurse turnover during the past 6 months; as a result, several new baccalaureate graduates work alongside seasoned nurses who have been practicing in the unit for more than 10 years. Although Derick is a new master's-prepared clinical nurse specialist for the unit, Trish does not think that he fully understands EBP given that he graduated from an academic program with a heavy research methods course in the curriculum and one that requires its students to complete a mini research proposal. Trish's interactions with and observations of the nurses delivering care over the past month lead her to conclude that there is a wide variation in their EBP knowledge and skills. However, this conclusion is based on her intuition and anecdotal evidence.

In reviewing the current issue of *Worldviews on Evidence-Based Nursing*, Trish sees a publication by Melnyk, Gallagher-Ford, Long, and Fineout-Overholt (2014) that outlines 13 new EBP competencies for practicing registered nurses (RNs) and an additional 11 competencies for advanced practice nurses (APNs). (Look ahead to Tables 2.1 and 2.2 to see these competencies.)

To be more evidence-based in her assessment of where the nurses are in terms of their EBP competency, Trish decides to use these competencies and asks her staff to respond to a questionnaire that asks whether they believe they are competent in each of the 13 items. In addition, Trish asks Derick to rate whether he is competent in the 13 competencies for practicing RNs along with the additional 11 for APNs.

As suspected, the data that Trish collected from the nurses in the ICU confirmed her suspicion that there was wide variance in the EBP competency of her staff. Derick believed he met 8 of the 13 competencies for practicing RNs and 5 of the 11 competencies for APNs. Therefore, Trish decided to send Derick to an intensive 5-day EBP immersion workshop offered by the Center for Transdisci-plinary EBP at The Ohio State University College of Nursing in order for him to gain the knowledge and skills needed to meet all 24 competencies and be able to fulfill the role of an EBP mentor for the ICU staff.

The assessment also allowed her and Derick to design and individualize an EBP continuing education program for each of the staff in her unit. For those staff members who reported that they felt competent in just a few of the 11 areas, they designed a comprehensive 6-month EBP fellowship program. For those who reported that they met the majority of the 11 EBP competencies, an abbreviated 2-month version of the EBP fellowship program was implemented. At the begin-ning of these two programs, Trish was clear in her communications with staff that she expected them to meet all 11 EBP competencies in order that their patients receive the highest quality of care. At the same time, she assured them that she would also "walk the talk" and make sure that they had the needed support and culture to consistently deliver EBP. Trish got her staff excited about the vision of being part of an "A" team that would be the lead unit in the hospital for EBP and having a reputation of best outcomes.

Within 2 years, every nurse met the 11 EBP competencies, and patient outcomes in the ICU were substantially improved. The ICU became a model for high-quality evidence-based care for the rest of the hospital. As a result, Trish was able to assist other nurse managers in implementing EBP programs and building a culture to ensure that their staff was competent in evidence-based care.

IMPORTANCE OF EVIDENCE-BASED PRACTICE COMPETENCIES

Competency is commonly defined as the capability to do something well. The American Nurses Association (2010, p. 64) has defined competency as "an expected and measurable level of nursing performance that integrates knowledge, skills, abilities, and judgment, based on established scientific knowledge and expectations for nursing practice." Dunn and colleagues (2000, p. 341) noted that competency is "not a skill or task to be done, but characteristics required in order to act effectively in the nursing setting." Competencies support the delivery of high-quality safe nursing care, which should be an expectation from the public (American Nurses Association, 2010; Melnyk et al., 2014).

The American Nurses Association (2010) has contended that no single evaluation or method can guarantee competence and also that it should be evaluated by the individual nurse (self-assessment), nurse peers, supervisors, and—in certain situations—patients. Measurement of nursing and other healthcare providers' competencies related to multiple patient care activities is an ongoing activity in multiple healthcare systems throughout the United States and the world.

Efforts to establish competencies for nursing pre-licensure and graduate education in order to prepare nurses to acquire the knowledge, skills, and attitudes to deliver safe, high-quality care have been part of the Quality and Safety Education for Nurses (QSEN) project (QSEN, 2013). The QSEN competencies, which are based on the Institute of Medicine (IOM) competency recommendations for healthcare professionals (IOM, 2003), address the following practice areas:

- Patient-centered care

- Teamwork and collaboration

- Evidence-based practice

- Quality improvement

- Safety

- Informatics

The definition of the QSEN competency for EBP is to integrate best current evidence with clinical expertise, family preferences, and values for delivery of optimal care (American Association of Colleges of Nursing QSEN Education Consortium, 2012). Evidence-based practice competencies for nursing education were developed by Stevens and colleagues to assist faculty in preparing their students for EBP and to "provide a basis for professional competencies in clinical practice" (Stevens, 2005, p. 8). However, a set of EBP research-based competencies had never been developed for practicing RNs and APNs in clinical settings. To fill a critical gap in nursing EBP competencies for practicing RNs and APNs, Melnyk and colleagues (2014) embarked on a two-step process to develop contemporary EBP competencies to assist healthcare organizations in ensuring that RNs and APNs are delivering the highest quality of evidence-based care.

Phase I: Development and Validation of the EBP Competencies

The competencies for practicing RNs and APNs were first drafted by Bernadette Melnyk and Ellen Fineout-Overholt, two nationally/internationally recognized experts in EBP with numerous years of experience facilitating healthcare systems and clinicians throughout the United States and world to advance and sustain EBP. Next, a panel of seven national experts from both academia and practice were convened via a series of teleconferences to review the drafted competencies and arrive at consensus regarding them. These experts were chosen because of their national reputation in EBP and extensive publications on the topic. Through a consensus-building validation process, the national panel came to consensus on 12 essential EBP competencies for practicing RNs and 11 additional EBP competencies for APNs.

Phase II: Validation of the EBP Competencies Through Research

The second phase of developing the final set of EBP competencies involved the conduct of a national Delphi study.

METHODS USED IN CONDUCTING A DELPHI STUDY

A *Delphi study* is a research method that uses experts to arrive at consensus through two or more structured rounds of a survey. Delphi studies use an iterative multistage process wherein experts are provided with feedback from the first round of the survey to consider in the next round of the survey. The process of surveying the experts is stopped when consensus is achieved, which usually takes two to three rounds (Hasson, Keeney, & McKenna, 2000).

Institutional review board approval by the authors' institution was granted for the Delphi study. The experts in the Delphi EBP survey were EBP mentors from across the U.S. who had attended an intensive EBP immersion workshop at the authors' academic institution during the previous 7 years. Each mentor was asked to respond to the following questions for each competency on a 5-point Likert scale that ranged from 0 (not at all) to 5 (very much so):

- To what extent do you believe the above EBP competency is essential for practicing registered professional nurses (or APNs, depending on the item)?

- Is the competency statement clearly written? If the mentors answered no to this second question, they were asked to rewrite the item.

The criterion for agreement was that 70% of the EBP mentors would rate each of the 23 EBP competencies between 4.5 and 5 on the 5-point Likert scale.

The initial request to participate in this study was sent to a database of 315 EBP mentors in July 2012. The potential subjects were provided information about the study and were informed that the completion of the survey gave their consent to participate in the research. The survey, which ran for 2 weeks, consisted of:

- Demographic questions

- Rating the 12 EBP competencies for practicing RNs

- Rating the 11 EBP competencies for APNs

Eighty EBP mentors responded to the first round of the Delphi study (a 25% participation rate). All EBP mentors who responded were female, with an average age of 52. They reported an average of 26 years of clinical practice experience, and the majority had master's or doctoral degrees and were currently serving in the EBP mentor role. Forty-five percent of the mentors worked in Magnet®-designated institutions.

In the first round of the survey (October 2012), each practicing RN and APN competency reached consensus in response to the first question (whether the competency is essential). However, four of the competencies for RNs were recommended for rewording and were rewritten based on the EBP mentors' feedback. In addition, it was recommended that one of those four RN competencies be split into two competencies, which meant that consensus needed to be obtained on these five newly worded RN competencies.

A second round of the survey was sent to the EBP mentors who completed the first round survey. Fifty-nine of the original 80 EBP mentors responded to the second survey (a 74% response rate) and rated the five reworded competencies for RNs. Total consensus was reached by the EBP mentors on the second round of the survey, which resulted in the final set of 13 EBP competencies for RNs and 11 additional competencies for APNs (Melnyk et al., 2014).

Remember that APNs need to be competent in the 13 competencies for RNs as well as the 11 competencies for APNs.

Table 2.1 lists the competencies for RNs and APNs; Table 2.2 lists the competencies dedicated to APNs.

TABLE 2.1 EVIDENCE-BASED PRACTICE COMPETENCIES FOR RNS AND APNS

Competency	Explanation
1	Questions clinical practices for the purpose of improving the quality of care.
2	Describes clinical problems using internal evidence.* (internal evidence*= evidence generated internally within a clinical setting, such as patient assessment data, outcomes management, and quality improvement data)
3	Participates in the formulation of clinical questions using PICOT* format. (*PICOT=Patient population; Intervention or area of Interest; Comparison intervention or group; Outcome; Time)
4	Systemically searches for external evidence* to answer focused clinical questions. (external evidence*= evidence generated from research)

continues

TABLE 2.1 EVIDENCE-BASED PRACTICE COMPETENCIES FOR RNS AND APNS   (CONTINUED)

Competency	Explanation
5	Participates in critical appraisal of pre-appraised evidence. (such as clinical practice guidelines, evidence-based policies and procedures, and evidence syntheses)
6	Participates in the critical appraisal of published research studies to determine their strength and applicability to clinical practice.
7	Participates in the evaluation and synthesis of a body of evidence gathered to determine its strength and applicability to clinical practice.
8	Collects practice data (e.g., individual patient data, quality improvement data) systematically as internal evidence for clinical decision-making in the care of individuals, groups, and populations.
9	Integrates evidence gathered from external and internal sources in order to plan evidence-based practice changes.
10	Implements practice changes based on evidence and clinical expertise and patient preferences to improve care processes and patient outcomes.
11	Evaluates outcomes of evidence-based decisions and practice changes for individuals, groups, and populations to determine best practices.
12	Disseminates best practices supported by evidence to improve quality of care and patient outcomes.
13	Participates in strategies to sustain an evidence-based practice culture.

TABLE 2.2 EVIDENCE-BASED PRACTICE COMPETENCIES FOR ADVANCED PRACTICE NURSES

Competency	Explanation
14	Systematically conducts an exhaustive search for external evidence* to answer clinical questions. (external evidence* = evidence generated from research)
15	Critically appraises relevant pre-appraised evidence (i.e., clinical guidelines, summaries, synopses, syntheses of relevant external evidence) and primary studies, including evaluation and synthesis.
16	Integrates a body of external evidence from nursing and related fields with internal evidence* in making decisions about patient care. (internal evidence*= evidence generated internally within a clinical setting, such as patient assessment data, outcomes management, and quality improvement data)
17	Leads transdisciplinary teams in applying synthesized evidence to initiate clinical decisions and practice changes to improve the health of individuals, groups, and populations.
18	Generates internal evidence through outcomes management and EBP implementation projects for the purpose of integrating best practices.
19	Measures processes and outcomes of evidence-based clinical decisions.
20	Formulates evidence-based policies and procedures.
21	Participates in the generation of external evidence with other healthcare professionals.
22	Mentors others in evidence-based decision-making and the EBP process.
23	Implements strategies to sustain an EBP culture.
24	Communicates best evidence to individuals, groups, colleagues, and policy makers.

Copyright 2016 The American Nurses Credentialing Center. Authors: Melnyk, B. M., Gallagher-Ford, L., & Fineout-Overholt, E.

IMPLICATIONS FOR USE OF THE EBP COMPETENCIES

The incorporation of these EBP competencies into the structure and operations of healthcare systems will enhance healthcare quality and patient outcomes as well as reduce costs. With a set of EBP competencies for practicing RNs and APNs in place, it is critical that they are used in healthcare systems across the United States to ensure high-quality nursing care. They also can be used in academic programs to ensure that RN and APN graduates are competent in EBP when they enter clinical settings.

In orientation/onboarding sessions for new nurses, an organizational vision and mission for EBP should be shared along with the EBP competencies. During this onboarding process, the expectation of achieving these competencies should be communicated. However, it must be realized that both RNs and APNs will enter the healthcare system with a wide variation in EBP knowledge and skills. Therefore, the competencies can be used immediately by having nurses rate themselves as to whether they meet each item. For those who believe that they are not competent in certain areas, EBP workshops and skills-building educational sessions can be held to assist them in achieving the competencies. Given that recognition is important to keep people motivated and engaged, an ongoing recognition program could be launched to highlight and recognize those nurses who achieve all EBP competencies.

Leaders and managers also should be held to the same expectation for meeting the competencies because if they do not "walk the talk" and be a role model for EBP, their staff will unlikely consistently deliver evidence-based care. Further, leaders and managers should create and support an EBP culture and environment with the necessary resources and tools for clinicians to succeed in delivering evidence-based care, including access to electronic databases for evidence searching and a critical mass of EBP mentors who work directly with point-of-care staff to implement EBP. Only with a supportive EBP culture and environment will evidence-based care thrive and sustain.

EBP competencies should also be written into job descriptions for RNs, APNs, and leaders/managers. During interviews for positions, candidates should be made aware of the expectation for EBP and also asked about their level of EBP knowledge and skills. The competencies also should be incorporated into performance evaluations as well as embedded into organizational policies and guideline development processes. Until all nurses achieve the EBP competencies, they should be embedded into clinical ladder programs as an incentive to become more skilled in EBP (Melnyk & Gallagher-Ford, 2015). A more comprehensive guide for implementing the EBP competencies in clinical settings can be found in Chapter 10.

SUMMARY

The development of research-based EBP competencies for practicing RNs and APNs is a major step in facilitating the delivery of high-quality, safe, and cost-effective care in hospitals and healthcare systems throughout the U.S. Healthcare organizations and academic programs should expect and provide the necessary supports for their nurses, APNs, and graduates to achieve these competencies in order to ensure the best outcomes for patients and their families.

REFERENCES

American Association of Colleges of Nursing (AACN) QSEN Education Consortium. (2012). *Graduate level QSEN competencies*. Washington, DC: AACN.

American Nurses Association. (2010). *Nursing. Scope and standards of practice* (2nd ed.). Washington, DC: American Nurses Association.

Dunn, S. V., Lawson, D., Robertson, S., Underwood, M., Clark, R., Valentine, T., & Herewane, D. (2000). The development of competency standards for specialist critical care nurses. *Journal of Advanced Nursing, 31*(2), 339–346.

Hasson, F., Keeney, S., & McKenna, H. (2000). Research guidelines for the Delphi survey technique. *Journal of Advanced Nursing, 32*(4), 1008–1015.

Institute of Medicine. (2003). Committee on Assuring the Health of the Public in the 21st Century. *The future of the public's health in the 21st century*. Washington, DC: National Academies Press.

Melnyk, B. M., & Gallagher-Ford, L. (2015). Implementing the new evidence-based practice competencies in real world clinical and academic settings: Moving from evidence to action in improving healthcare quality and patient outcomes. *Worldviews on Evidence-Based Nursing, 12*(2), 67–69.

Melnyk, B. M., Gallagher-Ford, L., & Fineout-Overholt, E. (2013) Evidence-based practice competencies for practicing registered nurses and advanced practice nurses. Columbus, Ohio: Authors.

Melnyk, B. M., Gallagher-Ford, L., Long, L., & Fineout-Overholt, E. (2014). The establishment of evidence-based
practice competencies for practicing nurses and advanced practice nurses in real-world clinical settings:
Proficiencies to improve healthcare quality, reliability, patient outcomes, and costs. *Worldviews on Evidence-
Based Nursing, 11*(1), 5–15.

Quality and Safety Education for Nurses (QSEN). (2013). Retrieved from http://qsen.org/about-qsen/project-
overview

Stevens, K. R. (2005). *Essential competencies for evidence-based practice in nursing* (1st ed.). San Antonio, TX:
Academic Center for Evidence-Based Practice, University of Texas Health Science Center.

ACHIEVING COMPETENCY WITH THE EVIDENCE-BASED PRACTICE COMPETENCIES

In Chapters 3–9, you learn markers of competence for each EBP competency as well as assessment strategies that facilitate implementation of the competencies in real-world clinical settings.

Chapter 3. 33

Chapter 4. 55

Chapter 5. 77

Chapter 6. 109

Chapter 7. 129

Chapter 8. 143

Chapter 9. 163

THE EVIDENCE-BASED PRACTICE COMPETENCIES RELATED TO CLINICAL INQUIRY

Lynn Gallagher-Ford, PhD, RN, DPFNAP, NE-BC

KEY CONTENT IN THIS CHAPTER

- Clinical inquiry defined and described

- Building a culture that supports clinical inquiry

- Evidence-based practice competencies #1, #2, and #3

- Strategies for building and promoting clinical inquiry

- Assessment of evidence-based practice (EBP) competencies related to clinical inquiry

- Implementing clinical inquiry competencies

> The important thing is not to stop questioning.
>
> –Albert Einstein

SETTING THE STAGE

Yamei is a staff nurse in the labor and delivery (L&D) unit of a large community hospital that delivers more than 2,500 babies annually. Yamei has been an L&D nurse for 17 years and is well respected by her peers and colleagues. Yamei is a strong advocate for skin-to-skin contact ("kangaroo care") for mothers and newborns as best practice, and her hospital provides skin-to-skin care for vaginally delivered babies and their mothers. Yamei recently attended a regional maternal-child consortium meeting and discovered that many hospitals had instituted skin-to-skin care for C-section patients, which was currently not the practice at her hospital because the anesthesiologists believed it was "unsafe to do in an OR setting." Yamei is very curious whether this practice has been shown to be safe for C-section patients. If so, what is the best way to offer it to patients (Step #0 in the EBP process).

Upon her return to work, Yamei contacts Colleen, the maternal-child health nurse educator, and shares her curiosity about offering skin-to-skin care to C-section patients. Colleen is excited that Yamei is interested in this question because it is something she also has questioned. Yamei and Colleen agree that they need help finding the evidence to answer their question, and they reach out to Rita, the EBP mentor in the education department. Rita meets with Yamei and Colleen and spends time with them clarifying the issue that they want to address. Rita works with Yamei and Colleen to formulate the best PICOT question (Step #1 in EBP) to help them with their search for external evidence to guide their practice change decision-making process.

They are interested in a wide range of outcomes that have been positively impacted by their skin-to-skin program with their non–C-section patients, including initial feeding time, breast feeding rates, infant temperature regulation, and patient satisfaction. Their EBP mentor encourages them to narrow their question to address the most important "so-what outcomes"—the ones that will help them make their case to stakeholders at their hospital. With the guidance of their EBP mentor, they develop the following PICOT question:

*In C-section patients (P), how does skin-to-skin care (kangaroo care) (I) com-
pared to traditional initial newborn care (C) affect initial feeding time (O) infant
temperature regulation (O) and patient satisfaction (O)?*

Based on the PICOT question, the team conducts an evidence search in the
Cochrane Database of Systematic Reviews, MEDLINE, and Cumulative Index to
Nursing and Allied Health Literature (CINAHL) and finds 11 studies that are
helpful in answering their question (Step #2 in EBP). With the help of their EBP
mentor, they critically appraise and synthesize the findings from the studies and
conclude that skin-to-skin care can be offered safely in the OR setting and that it
has been shown to positively affect all of the key outcomes they are interested in
(Step #3 in EBP). Based on the evidence, they provide the information to their key
stakeholders and work together to implement a limited test of this EBP change
with their low-risk C-section patients (Step #4 of the EBP process) before rolling
it out to a larger population. The limited rollout is well received; providers and
patients all offer positive feedback, and the patient outcomes are excellent (Step
#5 of the EBP process). Based on these results, the program is expanded and
becomes the standard of care for all new mothers and babies (unless an emergency situation overrides it). Yamei and Colleen, along with an obstetrician and an
anesthesiologist, present the EBP change project and results at a national OB/
GYN conference (Step #6 of the EBP process), where it is recognized as an excellent exemplar of transdisciplinary EBP.

CLINICAL INQUIRY DEFINED AND DESCRIBED

Melnyk and Fineout-Overholt (2015, p. 10) have defined *clinical inquiry* as a
"consistently questioning attitude toward practice": an ongoing curiosity about
best practices, and an inquisitiveness about the best evidence to guide clinical
decision-making (Melnyk & Fineout-Overholt, 2011). Clinical inquiry begins
with a state of mind and leads to specific behaviors that contribute to a culture of
EBP. As individuals and/or groups of nurses question current nursing practices,
they begin to recognize which of those practices might require change and learn
how they can make professional contributions to improve patient outcomes by
incorporating evidence into practice (Dogherty, Harrison, & Graham, 2010).

Clinical inquiry reflects an individual's ability to seek knowledge and/or identify clinical problems and issues. Most often, clinical inquiry is driven by practitioners' intellectual curiosity, their interest in ensuring that best practices are being used, and their desire that optimal clinical outcomes be achieved (Stillwell, Fineout-Overholt, Melnyk, & Williamson, 2010).

BUILDING A CULTURE THAT SUPPORTS CLINICAL INQUIRY

Clinical inquiry is Step #0 in the EBP process and, like EBP in general, can be either encouraged and nurtured or discouraged and discounted by peers, colleagues, and leaders. For clinical inquiry to begin and grow in an organization, it must be developed and nurtured in individuals. For clinical inquiry to thrive and become the norm of an organization, it also must be encouraged, acted upon, recognized, and celebrated. These activities require a culture and environment that is supportive of EBP overall, and leadership is essential to the development and sustainability of a culture of inquiry and EBP. Leaders must role-model inquiry themselves in their leadership practices; promote inquiry through creation of visible, accessible, and engaging structures; support inquiry through meaningful recognition and celebration; and, perhaps most importantly, publicly navigate barriers to inquiry.

Practice in many organizations is built on tradition and the embedded influence of sacred cows. The contemporary definition of a *sacred cow* is an individual, organization, or institution that is exempt from criticism or questioning. Practice and decision-making based in these constructs is often outdated and potentially harmful. Organizations and individuals must find ways to break away from these antiquated approaches in order to assure that current, best practice is delivered.

One example of an individual finding a way to break away from an antiquated approach is the Sacred Cow Contest. Introduced by Brown in 1993, it provided a creative strategy used to promote clinical inquiry. Brown conducted the Sacred Cow Contest to identify traditional nursing practices routinely carried out but not justified as best practices. Brown found that many nurses continued to practice according to how they were taught during their basic nursing education programs, whether they had graduated 3 or 30 years ago. Brown's Sacred Cow Contest provides a creative strategy to promote clinical inquiry and generate interest in EBP.

Another example of eliminating a sacred cow environment is when Mick (2011) replicated this strategy in a large healthcare system and inspired nurses to question traditional nursing practices. In Mick's organization, the Sacred Cow Contest increased discussion of EBP and generated interest in learning how to use the EBP process to answer clinical practice questions. As nurses examined practices and actions in their work setting, they began to identify many traditional practices that had no supporting rationale. Identification of sacred cows was a first step to resolving questionable practices. As sacred cows were reported, EBP workgroups identified relevant practice topics to explore to promote best nursing practices patient outcomes.

Clinical inquiry is a process that directly shifts decision-making to a scientific and reliable approach. The spirit of inquiry, where curiosity and ongoing questioning of practices, traditions, routines, and "the way we have always done it here" are the norm, underpins an evidence-based culture and eliminates sacred cows.

A culture that supports inquiry can be made visible in a variety of ways, such as:

- Inclusion of inquiry as a core value in organizational and departmental mission statements

- Development of organizational structures, such as job descriptions, onboarding programs, performance appraisals, and clinical promotion programs that reflect the expectation of ongoing clinical inquiry

- Provision of resources that support inquiry, such as PICOT boxes or whiteboards where questions can be collected

- Availability of a cadre of EBP mentors who are readily accessible and can partner with clinicians to articulate their clinical inquiry effectively

- Development of unit-based or organization-wide programs specifically designed to promote curiosity, wonder, and inquiry

The EBP competencies that address clinical inquiry are:

#1 Questions clinical practices for the purpose of improving the quality of care.

#2 Describes clinical problems using internal evidence.

#3 Participates in the formulation of clinical questions using PICOT (Patient population; Intervention or area of Interest; Comparison intervention or group; Outcome; Time) format. (See Chapter 1 for more about PICOT.)

When clinical inquiry is a required competency and expectation of practice, clinicians are accountable for asking questions that reflect:

- Current state of practice in a particular setting

- Needs of patients, clinicians, and staff

- Environmental factors affecting patients, clinicians, and staff

Clinical inquiry can be measured and evaluated. By including inquiry as a performance expectation, the individual clinician can be asked to delineate the questions they posed during the previous evaluation period and whether those questions led to EBP changes and improved outcomes.

COMPETENCY #1

Questions clinical practices for the purpose of improving the quality of care.

This competency is the basic and critical underpinning of the evidence-based clinician. Without questioning practice, the opportunities to improve practice are limited. Clinical questions rise out of day-to-day practice, regardless of position or specialty. Questions should be flowing from clinicians at every level as well as from their leaders. There is no formalized structure for asking a clinical question.

Some inquiries are very simple, such as, "Is turning patients every 2 hours the most effective nursing activity to prevent pressure ulcers?" Some inquiries are more complex and/or present themselves as stories, such as, "On our large medical-surgical unit, we have a lot of patients that are elderly who come in from nursing homes with long-standing indwelling catheters, and we also have a lot of surgical patients who come to us from the OR with a new catheter. Although we are working hard to get patients' catheters removed as fast as we can, our UTI rates are still higher than they should be, especially in patients with catheters. One of the reasons is that there is often a delay in getting an order from the attending physician to remove the catheter. We are wondering if there is a way to remove catheters more efficiently using a standing catheter removal protocol that is nurse-driven to see if we can decrease our CAUTI rates?" Either way, inquiry is the beginning of the EBP journey—and without inquiry, there is no EBP journey.

Strategies for Implementing Competency #1

- Integrate inquiry as a core value in the unit and/or departmental and/or organizational mission statement. See the sidebar for a nursing practice mission statement.

- Create the expectation that clinical inquiry is a competency and performance expectation. See the sidebar for an example of a registered nurse job description.

  - Include clinical inquiry content in onboarding programs.

  - Include clinical inquiry language in job descriptions and performance appraisal.

- Many clinicians in current practice never learned EBP, so education must be provided to build EBP knowledge and skills.

- EBP mentors should be easily accessible to point-of-care clinicians.

- The natural "knowledge brokers" in an organization (clinical nurse specialists, educators, and professional development practitioners) are excellent choices to develop/educate as EBP mentors.

- The EBP mentor role must be clearly articulated within the organization.

- EBP mentor job descriptions with specific EBP deliverables should be created. See the sidebar for an example of an EBP mentor job description.

- Development of a critical mass of EBP mentors, as first proposed in the Advancing Research and Clinical practice through close Collaboration (ARCC) model (Melnyk & Fineout-Overholt, 2002), is an effective strategy to promote inquiry and EBP. When a cadre of EBP mentors is made available to point-of-care clinicians throughout healthcare systems, they facilitate evidence-based care and improve patient outcomes (Melnyk, 2007; Levin, Fineout-Overholt, Melnyk, Barnes, & Vetter, 2011; Wallen et al., 2010).

- Use PICOT boxes.

  - PICOT boxes are a creative way of making the collection of clinical questions easy. They are simple boxes placed around a clinical area where clinicians can write what they are wondering about and drop their questions in the box. The questions are collected and reviewed on a regular basis. The questions obtained from front-line clinicians are then followed up by an EBP mentor or leader and used to begin the EBP process.

Different organizations have created a variety of processes to organize the questions, but the common theme is providing a place where questions can flow from point-of-care clinicians to the EBP mentors in the organization and, ultimately, to driving practice change.

- Implement fun and engaging programs to encourage inquiry. Figure 3.1 shows an example of an engaging PICOT activity—PICOT Bingo.

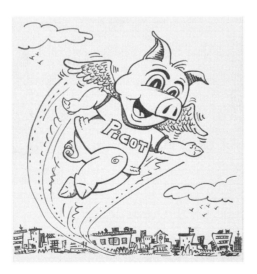

© Copyright October 2014
Tonya L. Smith, MSN, RN

Figure 3.1 PICOT Bingo.

A fun character (such as *PICOT the Flying Pig*) can be used to create interest in the idea of EBP, as shown in Figure 3.2. For example, the character could be used to decorate whiteboards, or PICOT boxes used to promote clinical inquiry.

FIGURE 3.2 Characters can be used to generate interest in EBP.

Copyright Lynn Gallagher-Ford. Artist; M. Gallagher; 2015

PROFESSIONAL NURSING PRACTICE MISSION

The professional practice of nursing combines scientific precision with empathy in caring for and nurturing of patients. Nurses thrive in *an environment that promotes clinical inquiry,* and inclusion of best evidence, clinical expertise, and patient voice to underpin our care....

See Chapter 10 for a complete nursing mission statement example.

Many organizations have created engaging programs to introduce and build EBP. These programs often include targeted strategies to promote inquiry. Introducing nonintimidating ways to be curious, ask questions, or wonder about what might be a better way to deliver care have been very effective in organizations of every size and level of complexity.

Assessment of Competency #1

Is the RN or APN able to:

- Express inquiry for the purpose of improving quality of care verbally or in writing.

- Clearly articulate clinical questions to improve quality of care.

- Use mechanisms to bring clinical questions forward appropriately.

- List the clinical questions that they have raised.

- Identify the impact of the questions they have brought forward on quality of care and outcomes.

REGISTERED NURSE JOB DESCRIPTION

- Establishes a compassionate environment by providing emotional, psychological, and spiritual support to patients, friends, and families
- Participates in EBP by questioning practices to improve care, describing clinical problems using evidence, participating in the steps of the EBP process, promoting a culture of EBP
- Participates in research activities when appropriate
- Promotes patient's independence by establishing patient care goals; teaching patient and family to understand condition, medications, and self-care skills; answering questions
- Assures quality of care by adhering to nursing ethics and standards; measuring health outcomes against patient care goals and standards; making evidence-based recommendations; following hospital and nursing division's philosophies and standards of care set by state board of nursing, state nurse practice act, and other governing agency regulations
- Resolves patient problems and needs by using multidisciplinary team strategies
- Promotes a safe and positive working environment
- Maintains continuity of care by documenting and communicating actions, irregularities, and continuing needs
- Maintains patient confidence and protects operations by keeping information confidential
- Maintains professional competence (knowledge, skills, and attitudes) by attending ongoing educational programs, reviewing professional publications, establishing personal networks, participating in professional organization(s)
- Communicates effectively with healthcare team members by active participation in clinical discussions, communicating information, responding to requests, building rapport, participating in team problem-solving

EBP MENTOR JOB DESCRIPTION

- Manages time effectively and is able to function independently and autonomously

- Facilitates a culture of EBP in nursing staff and other healthcare clinicians

- Coaches others in ongoing clinical inquiry

- Fosters critical thinking about clinical issues to encourage use of research findings in making clinical decisions

- Provides leadership for evidence-based projects, involving nurses and other transdisciplinary clinicians in the process

- Provides comprehensive EBP support to staff and colleagues, including formulating PICOT questions, conducting searches, evaluating and synthesizing a body of evidence, making recommendations for practice changes

- Navigates barriers to evidence-based care through active engagement with organizational leadership

- Collaborates with other healthcare providers in the integration of evidence in clinical decision-making

- Conducts EBP rounds to bring the latest research findings from studies to clinicians for implementation to improve patient outcomes

- Generates internal evidence through evidence-based quality improvement (QI) and outcomes management programs

- Participates in development of EBP guidelines, policies and procedures, standards, or practice models

- Provides leadership in attaining excellent clinical outcomes by acting as a communication link and consultant to providers and other caregivers across departments, campuses, or system

- Leads transdisciplinary teams in applying synthesized evidence to initiate clinical decisions and practice changes to improve the health of individuals, groups, and populations

- Coaches others in evidence-based clinical decision-making, patient/family education, and problem-solving

- Facilitates communication and promotes collaborative behavior among team members, including mentoring staff in effective communication techniques, conflict and crisis resolution, and team behaviors

- Participates in research activities when there is not sufficient evidence to address clinical issues

- Coordinates unit, multidepartment, or campus educational sessions in conjunction with educators, managers, and other experts

- Assists in creation of strategic learning plans related to EBP for staff

- Participates in multidepartment, campus, and/or system task forces or committees

- Teaches EBP courses or seminars at least twice per year or as needed

- Serves as a consultant to other departments related to EBP

- Actively participates in an outside professional organization to improve professional nursing practice

- Provides formal EBP–related presentations and/or posters at local or national venues

- Assists nursing staff in disseminating evidence through regional/national presentations and peer-reviewed journals

- Guides others in the Institutional Review Board (IRB) process

COMPETENCY #2

Describes clinical problems using internal evidence.* (internal evidence*= evidence generated internally within a clinical setting, such as patient assessment data, outcomes management, and quality improvement data)

The ability to express clinical questions in a way that reflects more than knee-jerk reactions to situations and anecdotal experience promotes a more efficient and meaningful EBP trajectory. When clinicians combine anecdotal experiences with data generated from their unit/organization, the data-supported inquiry is more likely to reflect the true issue or problem that is occurring. For this to be possible, point-of-care clinicians need to be made aware of and be oriented to sources of internal evidence on a given unit or within an organization. Clinicians should be given access to internal evidence sources so they can retrieve relevant data to support their inquiry. Openness and access to information is likely to promote and reinforce the spirit of inquiry amongst point-of-care clinicians. Clinicians will unlikely have the time and/or the patience to seek out internal evidence if it is held in remote locations and/or requires lengthy, cumbersome processes to acquire access.

 Remember that internal evidence is evidence generated internally within a clinical setting, such as patient assessment data, outcomes management, and quality improvement data.

Strategies for Implementing Competency #2

- Share internal unit-based and organizational evidence: for example, fall rates, catheter-associated urinary tract infection (CAUTI) rates, central line–associated bloodstream infection (CLABSI) rates, rehospitalization rates, patient satisfaction metrics, and so on with point-of-care clinicians on a regular basis.

- Provide point-of-care clinicians with access to internal evidence in open and welcoming ways.

- Help point-of-care clinicians in accessing and retrieving internal evidence.

- Mentor point-of-care clinicians in reading and understanding internal evidence documents (e.g., reports and spreadsheets).

Assessment of Competency #2

Is the RN or APN able to:

- Describe clinical problems using not only their anecdotal experiences, but also using evidence generated internally within their clinical setting.

- Articulate the internal evidence information that might be helpful in supporting the current clinical inquiry.

- Access internal evidence resources.

- Read and accurately describe the internal evidence being used.

  # COMPETENCY #3

Participates in the formulation of clinical questions using PICOT* format. (*PICOT=Patient population or other population; Intervention or area of Interest; Comparison intervention or group; Outcome; Time)

The formulation of a well-designed PICOT question is the critical step in the EBP process that takes a point-of-care clinician's clinical inquiry and converts it into a clear, concise question that can be used to effectively and efficiently search in electronic databases. In other words, a well-formulated PICOT question is the key to an effective and efficient search strategy. Many clinicians believe that a PICOT question is the "title" for their EBP project, but it is not. Instead, the literature that the PICOT question leads you to will define, inform, and shape your EBP project. Many clinicians want to change their PICOT question after they have completed their search because the search led them to additional information and evidence (i.e., down a path of which they were not expecting). That is exactly the function of the PICOT question—to take the clinician to all the literature that may answer his or her question, not just what the clinician thought was the answer.

 PICOT questions should never be changed: They should simply be retained as the part of the EBP process that led to the literature/evidence found.

However, once the function of the PICOT question is understood, it is quite simple: The PICOT question drives your search; it is not the title of your EBP project.

 Formulating a PICOT question requires that the clinician be able to identify key aspects of the situation:

P: Population

I: Intervention or Interest area

C: Comparison intervention if applicable

O: Outcome(s) that are expected to be impacted

T: Time (if appropriate)

Formulating a well-built PICOT question requires including terms that are likely to be found in the literature. In other words, local terms and abbreviations, such as "Dr. Smith's Pitocin protocol," "ABC Medical Center's fall prevention program," or "SCDs" should be avoided because they will not be found in the searchable databases. Generic and or generally accepted terminology and terms should be used in a PICOT question.

Formulating a PICOT question using a template makes it much easier to avoid making a mistake, such as using a direction in a PICOT question (increase, improve, promote), which could lead to a biased search or developing a research question inadvertently. The keywords arrived at through the PICOT process become the terms that will be used when searching the databases. Arriving at a clear articulation of these terms takes time and can often be facilitated by discussion with colleagues. For example, if you are wondering whether simulation is an effective way to teach nurses how to manage postpartum hemorrhage, the original question might be, "Is simulation an effective way to teach nurses how to manage postpartum hemorrhage?" This question could lead to a very ineffective search. By creating the following PICOT question, the key search terms become clearly articulated and are more likely to yield an effective search process that answers the question:

In nurses (P), how does simulation (I) compared to didactic lecture (C) affect knowledge acquisition (O)?

Formulating a perfect PICOT question on the first iteration is rarely possible. Discuss your clinical inquiry with peers and EBP mentors to clarify it before you start to draft your PICOT question. In addition to talking it over with colleagues, write your PICOT question draft and have others provide constructive feedback. These steps may take a few minutes upfront in the process, but they will save time in the long run because the better formulated your PICOT question, the better your search will be.

Strategies for Implementing Competency #3

- Educate clinicians about how to formulate effective PICOT questions.

- Educate clinicians about the purpose of the PICOT question (i.e., to drive the literature search).

- Mentor clinicians in formulating PICOT questions because it is a learned skill and requires practice.

- Use PICOT templates to guide formulation of effective PICOT questions. See Figure 3.3 for a template.

Assessment of Competency #3

Is the RN or APN able to:

- Describe the purpose of a PICOT question (i.e., to drive an effective and efficient literature search).

- Identify key aspects of the situation they are wondering about.

- Articulate generic and/or generally accepted terminology and terms in creating their PICOT.

- Integrate feedback to improve PICOT questions.

- Formulate a PICOT question that leads to an effective search process.

Templates for Asking Clinical Questions

INTERVENTION/THERAPY

In _____ (P), how does _____ (I) compared to _____ (C)

affect _____ (O) within _____ (T)?

PROGNOSIS/PREDICTION

In _____ (P), how does _____ (I) compared to _____ (C)

influence _____ (O) over _____ (T)?

DIAGNOSIS OR DIAGNOSTIC TEST

In _____ (P) are/is _____ (I) compared to _____ (C)

more accurate in diagnosing _____ (O)?

ETIOLOGY

Are_____ (P), who have _____ (I) compared to those

without _____ (C) at _____ risk for/of _____ (O)

over _____ (T)?

MEANING

How do _____ (P) with _____ (I) perceive _____ (O)

during _____ (T)?

Short definitions of different types of questions

Intervention/Therapy: Questions addressing the treatment of an illness or disability

Prognosis/Prediction: Questions addressing the prediction of the course of a disease

Diagnosis: Questions addressing the act or process of identifying or determining the nature and cause of a disease or injury through evaluation

Etiology: Questions addressing the causes or origins of disease (i.e., factors that produce or predispose toward a certain disease or disorder)

Meaning: Questions addressing how one experiences a phenomenon

FIGURE 3.3 PICOT question templates.

A REAL-WORLD EXAMPLE

MEETING COMPETENCIES #1, #2, AND #3

Tami is a staff nurse in the emergency department (ED) of a children's hospital that is affiliated with large medical and nursing schools. The ED is a very busy place, with a variety of students, residents, and fellows rotating through the department. The attending physicians and advanced practice providers in the department are quite experienced, and most are on the faculty of the medical school. Tami has worked with the ED team for 10 years and has developed strong and respectful relationships with everyone. In the past year, she has noticed variation in how children with acute asthma are being managed in the ED. Some providers have continued to order traditional nebulizer treatments, while others have begun to order asthma treatments using metered dose inhalers (MDIs) and spacers. Tami is wondering which of these treatments is best for their patients. Some of her questions include: Which treatment modality works faster?; Which treatment modality is tolerated better?; Which treatment modality has the least side effects?; and Is one treatment modality better than the other in terms of preventing hospitalization? (Step #0 in EBP).

Tami shares her curiosity with some of her colleagues and discovers that many of them have been wondering the same things. They discuss the current situation, sharing what they have experienced and observed anecdotally (internal evidence). Tami decides to take the questions forward in order to determine the best practice for their ED patients. Tami reaches out to her manager and the clinical nurse specialist (CNS) in the ED, who are both EBP mentors, and shares the list of questions posed by the ED staff. The manager and the CNS acknowledge that they also have recently noticed this variation in practice and feel it is an important set of questions to answer. Tami and her manager, along with the ED CNS, work together to develop several PICOT questions based on the general questions (clinical inquiry) that the ED staff group has articulated. Tami learns from her EBP mentors that using the PICOT question format is a technique that helps take general curiosity about an issue (i.e., clinical inquiry)

continues

continued

and generates questions that are well suited for performing literature searches in electronic databases.

Together, Tami and the EBP mentors from the ED develop the following PICOT questions (Step #1 in EBP):

- In children treated for acute asthma in the ED (P), how does a bronchodilator delivered by nebulizer (I) compared to an MDI and spacer (C) affect length of stay (O) while hospitalized (T)?

- In children treated for acute asthma in the ED (P), how does a bronchodilator delivered by nebulizer (I) compared to an MDI and spacer (C) affect the number and severity of treatment-related side effects (O)?

After Tami and the ED mentors have their PICOT questions formulated, they make an appointment to meet with the hospital librarian to begin the next step in the EBP process: searching for the best evidence to answer their questions (Step #2 in EBP). We discuss Step #2 in Chapter 4.

SUMMARY

Clinical inquiry is a critical underpinning of the entire EBP process. It is a state of mind that must be developed and nurtured in every clinician and cultural norm that must be developed and embedded in every organization. A culture of clinical inquiry means ongoing curiosity about best practices is expected and normal; it is not marginalized or unusual. When this state is achieved, an evidence-based approach to decision-making and practice is possible, and ultimately outcomes improve for patients, clinicians, and organizations.

REFERENCES

Dogherty, E., Harrison M., & Graham, I. (2010). Facilitation as a role and process in achieving evidence-based practice in nursing: A focused review of concept and meaning. *Worldviews on Evidence-Based Nursing, 7*(2), 76–89.

Levin, R., Fineout-Overholt, E., Melnyk, B., Barnes, M., & Vetter, M. J. (2011). Fostering evidence-based practice to improve nurse and cost outcomes in a community health setting: A pilot test of the advancing research and clinical practice through close collaboration model. *Nursing Administration Quarterly, 35*(1), 21–33. doi:10.1097/NAQ.0b013e31820320ff

Melnyk, B. (2007). The evidence-based practice mentor: A promising strategy for implementing and sustaining EBP in healthcare systems. *Worldviews on Evidence-Based Nursing, 4*(3), 123–125.

Melnyk, B. M., & Fineout-Overholt, E. (2002). Putting research into practice. Rochester ARCC. *Reflections on Nursing Leadership, 28*(2), 22–25.

Melnyk, B. M., & Fineout-Overholt, E. (2011). *Evidence-based practice in nursing & healthcare: A guide to best practice* (2nd ed.). Philadelphia, PA: Wolters Kluwer Lippincott Williams & Wilkins. Inova Health Sciences Library Call #: WY 100.7 M5 2011.

Melnyk, B. M., Gallagher Ford, L., Long, L. E., & Fineout-Overholt, E. (2014). The establishment of evidence-based practice competencies for practicing registered nurses and advanced practice nurses in real-world clinical settings: Proficiencies to improve healthcare quality, reliability, patient outcomes, and costs. *Worldviews on Evidence-Based Nursing, 11*(1), 5–15.

Melnyk, B. M., & Fineout-Overholt, E. (2015). *Evidence-based practice in nursing & healthcare: A guide to best practice* (3rd ed.). Philadelphia, PA: Wolters Kluwer.

Mick, J. (2011). Promoting clinical inquiry and evidence-based practice. *Journal of Nursing Administration, 41*(6), 280–284.

Stillwell, S., Fineout-Overholt, E., Melnyk, B., & Williamson, K. (2010). Evidence-based practice, step by step: Asking the clinical question: A key step in evidence-based practice. *American Journal of Nursing, 110*(3), 58–61.

Wallen, G., Mitchell, S., Melnyk, B., Fineout-Overholt, E., Miller-Davis, C., Yates, J., & Hastings, C. (2010). Implementing evidence-based practice: Effectiveness of a structured multifaceted mentorship programme. *Journal of Advanced Nursing, 66*(12), 2261–2277.

THE EVIDENCE-BASED PRACTICE COMPETENCIES RELATED TO SEARCHING FOR BEST EVIDENCE

Tami A. Hartzell, MLS, and
Ellen Fineout-Overholt, PhD, RN, FNAP, FAAN

KEY CONTENT IN THIS CHAPTER

- Constructing a basic strategy for systematic searching to answer clinical questions using PICOT format

- Evidence-based practice (EBP) competencies #4 and #14

- Advanced search strategy

- Organizing citations

- Locating grey literature

- Evaluation of systematic searching skills

> 'Data! Data! Data!' he cried impatiently. 'I can't make bricks without clay.'
>
> –Sherlock Holmes, The Adventure of the Copper Beeches

SETTING THE STAGE

Sheila is a bedside nurse primarily stationed on a surgical unit. She enjoys floating to other units and has recently been assigned to a vascular unit. She notices that the vascular unit patients are not walking as much as the patients on the surgical unit, and she wonders why. The literature she is aware of promotes ambulation as one intervention to accelerate recovery. When she asks a colleague why he doesn't have his patients walking more, she is told that bed rest is important for patients recovering from thrombotic events. Because Sheila knows that immobilization decreases muscle mass and strength, she wonders whether bed rest is really the appropriate strategy (Step #0 in EBP) for managing patients who are suffering from deep vein thrombosis (DVT) or pulmonary embolism (PE). She decides that a quick review of the literature is in order to satisfy her curiosity and formulates her PICOT question (Step #1 in EBP):

In patients hospitalized with PE or DVT (P), how does ambulation (I) compared to bed rest (C) affect rate of recovery (i.e., length of stay) (O) over one month (T)?

Sheila contemplates which sources to search that will give her the best answer. She determines that Cumulative Index to Nursing and Allied Health Literature (CINAHL), MEDLINE, and Cochrane Library are the most likely databases that will help her find the answer. She next thinks about what search approach to use across those databases. Using a PICOT worksheet to help guide her strategy, she fleshes out the terms she will search and begins her systematic search for evidence (Step #2 in EBP). Appendix A includes the *PICOT Worksheet and Search Strategy Development.*

Using keyword terms from her PICOT question and following the systematic approach, Sheila quickly finds several studies that address her question, including a systematic review and meta-analysis. After further discussion with some of her colleagues about the evidence she has found, she realizes that she has stumbled upon a "sacred cow" within the unit. Even though she found high-level, well-done evidence, she knows she will need to expand her search to look for more evidence because sacred cows require a well-constructed evidence synthesis to demonstrate the need for practice change. She also realizes that she must make good use of internal evidence from existing unit outcome data and begins conversations with the population-based advanced practice nurse (APN), who also is an EBP mentor, about how to work with the organizational processes to incorporate internal data into the EBP process.

Sheila and the EBP mentor quickly scan for subject headings as they review the citations found in performing the systematic search, and they realize it would be beneficial to include the subject headings *early ambulation*, *venous thrombosis*, *pulmonary embolism*, and *venous thromboembolism*. They decide to use *mobilization* as well, which is a synonym for ambulation, and the EBP mentor suggests also using the British spelling *mobilisation*. Restructuring Sheila's initial search strategy, they add subject headings and search again across all three databases she originally identified. More studies are found that will help Sheila present her case. After critically appraising the studies (Step #3 in EBP), the EBP mentor suggests that the nurses on the vascular unit also may respond well to an existing guideline for reducing PE or DVT risk for hospitalized patients. They search both Turning Research Into Practice (TRIP) and the National Guideline Clearinghouse and locate two guidelines: a recently revised guideline by the National Institute for Health and Care Excellence (2015) and an earlier one by the American College of Chest Physicians (2012). Both guidelines contain an ambulation recommendation that agrees with the evidence found in the systematic search.

Sheila asks her nurse manager when she can present the evidence to her colleagues. She and the EBP mentor prepare the presentation that includes the evidence synthesis and the internal evidence from the unit to share at the next staff meeting. While initially doubtful that ambulation is an intervention that will help their patients, the internal evidence demonstrated that length of stay is longer on their unit than the national average. Sheila's colleagues begin a discussion about the merits of ambulation in their patient population as outlined in the evidence synthesis. The staff decide that a team should develop unit-specific recommendations for ambulation from the evidence synthesis that they will implement on their floor over the next 6 months. Sheila is excited to head the team, and the team develops an ambulation protocol based on the evidence synthesis she and the EBP mentor put together. The team submits an *Evidence-Based Practice and*

Performance Improvement Project Form to the EBP & Quality Council for review as an evidence implementation project. The EBP & Quality Council provides permission to translate the evidence into practice, and the team presents the protocol rollout at the next staff meeting (Step #4 in EBP). The staff express excitement about implementing the protocol.

Across the next 6 months, the team reports at each staff meeting on the outcomes they have collected. At the end of the 6 months, the team reports that, as the evidence indicated, ambulation was not associated with a higher risk of developing a PE and that patients on the protocol did not develop a new thrombus. Furthermore, their existing DVT did not progress, and they were released sooner (Step #5 in EBP). Sheila and her team are excited about their results and share their findings at the hospital-wide Nursing Practice Council. They also submit an abstract to present at the hospital's research conference the following year. With additional encouragement from the EBP mentor, they develop a poster to present at the Society of Vascular Nursing regional meeting (Step #6 in the EBP process). Sheila would not have been able to make her case and change patient care had she not used a systematic approach for searching multiple databases to ensure that the resulting evidence base was relevant to her clinical question and guided the necessary practice improvement and subsequent outcomes.

DEVELOPING A SYSTEMATIC APPROACH TO SEARCHING

Evidence-based practice (EBP) calls for a systematic approach to searching multiple databases to ensure that the resulting evidence is relevant at the point when the search was completed. Systematically locating relevant evidence to guide nursing practice and improve patient care is an important skill that both registered nurses (RNs) and advanced practice nurses (APNs) need to master. The National Academy of Medicine's (formerly the Institute of Medicine) vision holds that by the year 2020, 90% of clinical decisions should be supported by accurate and up-to-date clinical information (IOM, 2009). At the same time, consumers are becoming more health-literate, and many expect to take an active role in their healthcare. Nurses need to ensure they are able to competently conduct a systematic search for the best evidence to answer patient questions as well as their own well-formulated PICOT question (see Competency #3, discussed in Chapter 3).

In the past, searching for evidence has been considered an "as you like it" activity. Often the steps and strategies for searching included thinking of the terms you wanted to search, putting the terms in the search box with Boolean AND or OR operators, and seeing what you found. The expectation was that whatever you found was fine—just bring it to the discussion. Wherever this approach to searching for (and retrieving) evidence is used, the results often lead to irrelevant articles. Furthermore, there is a tendency to search only one database. For nursing, it is the CINAHL database. This approach to searching can be frustrating when the yield is not what is needed. Furthermore, more time is invested in this approach to searching than with the streamlined, focused systematic approach.

Both RNs and APNs must have foundational searching skills that enable them to be competent at the basic level (see Table 4.1, Competency #4) (Melnyk, Gallagher-Ford, Long, & Fineout-Overholt, 2014). Advanced practice nurses must have advanced skills that enable them to perform an exhaustive search that leads to retrieving a greater amount of evidence through accessing a variety of sources of evidence in addition to the indexed healthcare databases (see Table 4.1, Competency #14) (Melnyk et al., 2014).

> In the past, searching for evidence has been considered an "as you like it" activity. Evidence-based practice (EBP) calls for a *systematic* approach to searching multiple databases to ensure that the resulting evidence is relevant at the point when the search was completed.

TABLE 4.1 SEARCH STRATEGY BEHAVIORS

Behavior	RN Competency #4	APN Competency #14
Determines search terms by		
Identifying main topics as well as terms/phrases through a well-developed PICOT question[a]	X	X
Determines appropriate databases or resources to search by		
Demonstrating familiarity with library resources to identify best sources to search[a,b,c]	X	X
Identifying open access (free) databases/resources to search[b]	X	X
Requesting assistance from librarian whenever necessary[b,c]	X	X
Constructs appropriate search strategy by		
Viewing instructional videos from database providers to master searching skills[c]	X	X
Using keyword searching[b,c]	X	X
Identifying controlled vocabulary and correctly applying it to search strategy[a,b,c]	X	X
Using Boolean (logic) operators correctly[a,b]	X	X
Executing advanced search features, such as adjacency and truncation[b]	X	X
Expanding search through use of subject headings, additional synonyms, explode commands, going further back in time[b,c]	X	X
Using limiters such as focus/major concept, population, language, age, publication type, gender, and publication date when necessary[a,b]	X	X
Consulting librarian for additional assistance with search strategy when necessary[b,c]	X	X

Searching a minimum of two databases/resources	X	X
Identifying additional concepts related to the original PICOT question		X
Expanding search by including British spelling variations, e.g. haematology, to increase yield[a]		X
Identifying grey literature, experts in the field, internal evidence[b]		X
Selects appropriate evidence to read by		
Selecting articles that most closely match PICOT question[b]	X	X
Selecting best available evidence using evidence hierarchy when applicable	X	X
Organizes citations and search strategies by		
Printing and/or saving list of citations (bibliography) and saving search history[b]	X	X
Using reference managers (such as Zotero or RefWorks) to organize citations or generate formatted bibliography and/or manuscript[b,c]		X
Obtains appropriate literature by		
Printing and/or downloading appropriate articles from databases	X	X
Using alternative sources to obtain copies of articles, such as the Internet or other libraries[a,b]	X	X
Printing and/or saving search strategies used during database searching	X	X
Using bibliography of keeper articles to locate additional articles that match PICOT question	X	X

continues

TABLE 4.1 SEARCH STRATEGY BEHAVIORS   (CONTINUED)

Behavior	RN Competency #4	APN Competency #14
Identifies and searches grey literature by		
Identifying appropriate associations and/or websites to search[a,b]		X
Identifying listservs that may be useful and initiates a post		X
Identifying internal/external evidence outside the realm of databases		X

[a]*Eldredge, Hendrix, & Karcher (2006)*

[b]*Hartzell, Fineout-Overholt, Hofstetter, & Ponder (2014)*

[c]*Technology Informatics Guiding Education Reform (TIGER) (2006)*

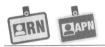

COMPETENCY #4

Systematically searches for external evidence* to answer focused clinical questions. (external evidence*= evidence generated from research)

Strategies for Implementing Competency #4

For Competency #4, every RN should be able to learn and implement these basic searching strategies in a systematic, sequential order:

1. **Determine search terms from the PICOT question.**

   - *Strategy 1:* Think about how to structure your search so you are consistent in your search approach across all databases searched. Take the terms you honed in the PICOT question and write them down along with other synonyms that may be associated with those topics. To help you organize your basic search, consider using the *PICOT Worksheet and Search Strategy Development* in Appendix A.

- *Strategy 2:* Determine the kind of evidence (research design, such as randomized controlled trials, systematic reviews, cohort studies) you are searching for, as this will help with your systematic approach (Hartzell et al., 2014).

2. Determine appropriate databases or resources to search (at least two).

- *Strategy 1:* Determine which databases contain articles/resources that will best answer your PICOT question. This requires some knowledge of what is offered by various healthcare databases. The databases most clinicians use in academic settings are *bibliographic,* meaning they contain journal article citations (e.g., CINAHL). Other databases used in clinical settings contain evidence summaries (e.g., EBSCO Nursing Reference Center). Generally, an evidence summary will highlight available evidence and provide recommendations for patient care.

- *Strategy 2:* Know which resources are available so you can select the best databases to search. If you are affiliated with a university or hospital, make sure you know what databases the library offers. If you are not affiliated with a university or hospital, check out the databases your local library provides related to healthcare. Several databases are free. PubMed and the TRIP database are among the best known (Hartzell et al., 2014).

  Google and Google Scholar also may be good sources to use, provided that you search appropriately (Younger, 2010). Recent studies have concluded that both Google and Google Scholar are effective in identifying relevant research (Kim et al., 2014; Nourbakhsh, Nugent, Wang, Cevik, & Nugent, 2012). However, Google Scholar should not be the only source you search. Make sure you use other healthcare databases, too.

3. Construct appropriate basic search strategy.

- *Strategy 1:* Learn to effectively search each database to save you time and frustration. Tutorials are available for most databases.

- *Strategy 2:* Select a database and begin your search. If available, use the advanced search feature and search in the title of the article for the outcome "O" term in your PICOT question. This initial step can help retrieve focused articles on the outcome (O) you have identified. Keywords appearing in the title of articles will probably be the article's main point.

- *Strategy 3:* Note the subject headings that were used to index the articles you just found and then search with those and any other appropriate subject headings. Use the focus features (MEDLINE) or the major concept feature (CINAHL) to ensure that the topic of interest is the main point of the articles retrieved.

- *Strategy 4:* Repeat Step 3 Strategies 1–3 for all terms within the PICOT question.

- *Strategy 5:* Combine the keywords and/or subject headings searches using the appropriate Boolean connector (also called logic operators): OR enables you to explore what is available with any of the terms (e.g., OR all the terms or subject headings within a single PICOT element); AND is used to ensure that all the terms in the PICOT question are present in the articles for which you are searching.

4. Select appropriate evidence to read.

- *Strategy 1:* Limit your results to establish a number of articles that you can manage after you have used the major concept feature.

- *Strategy 2:* Examine the set of article citations. This is the first step in including or excluding articles that match or don't match your PICOT question.

- *Strategy 3:* Actively think about the hierarchy/levels of evidence so that you spend your time wisely. For example, do you really want to spend time reading an editorial when you could spend it reading a systematic review or perusing a clinical trial, if they are available?

5. Obtain articles.

- *Strategy 1*: Locate a copy of the articles/studies you have selected for critical appraisal. Know how to print the full text articles that are available within the database. Some full text articles are immediately available within the database you are searching. For articles that are not available directly within the database, ask your favorite librarian to help you obtain a copy using interlibrary loan or search Google or Google Scholar. Also remember that public libraries can help provide you with articles that you have found through your searching. Just make sure you have the complete citation. If you have any questions, seek out a librarian.

- *Strategy 2:* Scan the reference lists of the articles that you have identified as appropriate for appraisal. Often this technique will yield additional articles that you have not identified in the database search.

- *Strategy 3:* Describe how you searched, how many potential articles you found, and how many you kept (see the upcoming sidebar for the short steps for a systematic search).

SHORT STEPS TO SEARCHING COMPETENTLY

Before your search:

- Start thinking about keywords from the PICOT question: the P, I, C, O, T.

- Be sure to click on Advanced Search if you aren't already in that mode.

- After you are in Advanced Search mode, follow these steps:

  1. Begin with the keyword for the outcome you wish to see occur/ change (O).

  2. If you have the opportunity to ask for subject headings, use that option.

continues

continued

3. Choose the subject heading *(controlled vocabulary)* that **best** fits your keywords. (MeSH is MEDLINE/PubMed's subject headings/controlled vocabulary.)

4. Choose explode, when available, to be sure to capture all the terms associated with the subject heading you have chosen, and also use the major concept feature to capture those articles with your subject heading as the main topic of the article.

5. Perform the search.

6. In CINAHL, be sure you click Search History (under the search boxes) so that you can see your search.

7. Enter each keyword/subject heading combination individually. Combine your searches for an individual PICOT element with OR. Look for the terms for which there are few articles and for which terms there are many articles. (Caveat: Clear the search box in CINAHL before each new search and before combining searches.)

8. After searching for each keyword/subject heading in PICOT, begin to combine the searches using AND.

9. When the AND search of all the PICOT elements brings a small yield, begin to combine systematically, starting with the O and I.

10. Continue to combine until you get a meaningful combined search that can best address your clinical question.

11. Describe what your final yield was in the current database in which you are searching and then across all databases you have searched. (See the *PICOT Worksheet and Search Strategy Development* in Appendix A.)

Assessment of Competency #4

Is the RN or APN able to:

- Demonstrate basic strategy for a systematic search within an Objective Structured Clinical Examination (OSCE).

- Successfully complete a quiz for knowledge of systematic searching technique and order of search strategy.

- Submit a screenshot or printed copy that demonstrates basic systematic searching techniques (see Figure 4.1).

- Submit a screenshot or printed copy of search for each database used.

- Demonstrate improvements in skills in systematic searching on annual performance evaluation.

COMPETENCY #14

Systematically conducts an exhaustive search for external evidence* to answer clinical questions. (external evidence* = evidence generated from research)

Strategies for Implementing Competency #14

Advanced practice nurses have basic searching skills as well as advanced searching skills. This is why some steps in this competency begin where the basic search left off. In addition, basic steps that have no advanced strategies are not listed. Advanced practice nurses, as advanced searchers, also are able to provide further guidance for basic searchers and delve deeper into the existing evidence.

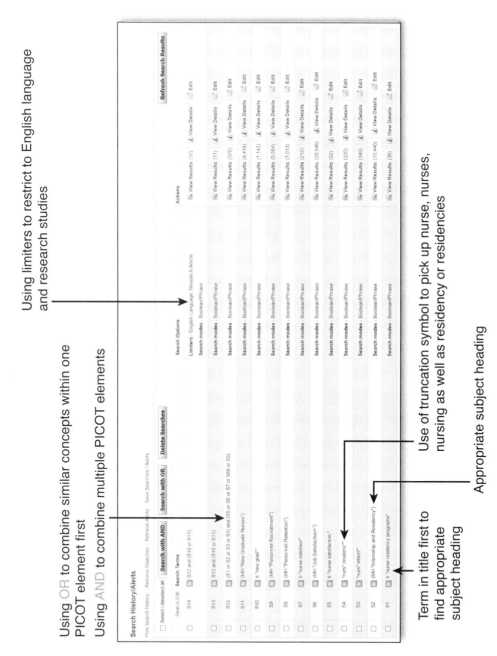

Figure 4.1   Sample search strategy.

3. Perform additional advanced strategies.

Remember that these steps leave off where the basic search strategies end, so this step list starts with Step 3.

- *Strategy 6:* Expand your search to find more articles:

    - Try additional synonyms or related concepts to the keywords.

    - Identify additional concepts related to the original PICOT question. For example, if you are working on a hearing amplifier protocol, also look for articles on treating or identifying cerumen impaction. In addition, further exploration can be achieved using the Boolean connector OR to pull together the terms or subject headings that are similar within each element of PICOT. That way, all citations that contain any of the terms or subject headings you are searching for will be retrieved.

    - Use adjacency (proximity) to retrieve more focused citations and truncation to retrieve additional citations.

    - Explode subject headings/MeSH terms.

    - Consider using British spelling variations such as paediatrics.

    - Go further back in time.

- *Strategy 7:* Apply limits to your search if you have too many articles:

    - Limit your search to articles written in or translated to English.

    - Limit by date of publication. Keep in mind that limiting the publication date may exclude some landmark works that were published outside the date range you have specified.

    - Limit by publication type. Think about the hierarchy of evidence and limit to randomized controlled trials or systematic reviews when applicable.

- *Strategy 8:* Identify additional sources that might be searched/consulted to answer the clinical question:

  - Grey literature

  - Librarians or other colleagues who are proficient in searching

  - Identified experts in the field

  - Internal evidence

4. Take additional advanced actions.

- *Strategy 5:* Print the list of articles you will be appraising. It's always favorable to have a complete list of the articles you think are relevant to the PICOT. Each database has a way to select and print those articles.

- *Strategy 6:* Print the screen capture or print a copy of your search strategy. Printing screen captures will be computer-dependent. Refer to your computer manual about this procedure or search Google to find how to accomplish this. Also, each database has a way to print out a copy of the search strategy. You will want a copy so that you can keep your search of other databases consist with the current search strategy.

5. Organize citations and search strategies.

- *Strategy 1:* Save the results of the search once the best articles/studies have been selected.

- *Strategy 2:* Document your search strategy so that you can replicate it across other databases at another time. This will also inform others about the search strategy you used (i.e., where and how you searched) and also allows you to organize your search results to maximize the use of the body of evidence.

- *Strategy 3:* Save your search strategy within the database (check the database help for how to do this) to allow returning to that same strategy so that you can run that strategy without having to reconstruct it.

- *Strategy 4:* Save your search strategy as an alert (check the database help for how to do this) so that you can have the most current citations forwarded to your email on a regular basis.

- *Strategy 5:* Use reference managers such as Zotero, Mendeley, EndNote, or RefWorks to help organize the search results and share them with your teams. Often with change, evidence-based quality improvement, and research projects, APNs must save the results of the search after the best articles/studies have been selected. Search Google for more information on these reference managers and others.

6. Find nonjournal literature (grey literature).

- *Strategy 1:* Complete comprehensive (i.e., exhaustive) searches to answer either your own APN PICOT questions or your team's questions. This approach requires APNs to search for unpublished studies as well as information from professional organizations, such as conference proceedings and guidelines.

- *Strategy 2:* Identify nursing associations, such as the Association of peri-Operative Registered Nurses (AORN), or other associations such as the American Cancer Society, and search their websites for relevant studies or guidelines whenever appropriate.

- *Strategy 3:* Seek help from colleagues and friends. Consider posting a question on an association listserv, for example, as other clinicians may have had the same question and could be quite willing to talk about the evidence they found.

Assessment of Competency #14

Is the APN able to:

- Submit a screenshot or printed copy that demonstrates advanced searching techniques with steps/strategies of a systematic search (refer to Figure 4.1).

- Demonstrate use of reference manager software (i.e., review contents and organization within the reference manager and how these contents would be shared with others).

- Demonstrate on annual performance evaluation improvements in skills in advanced searching.

REAL-WORLD EXAMPLE

MEETING COMPETENCIES #4 AND #14

Joanna is a doctorally prepared nurse practitioner working with Heidi, an RN, in a private internal medicine office. One of their patients has irritable bowel syndrome (IBS) and is suffering from recurrent clostridium difficile (C. Diff). On her latest visit, the patient asks Heidi whether she has heard of fecal transplants and wonders whether this treatment option might help her overcome her C. Diff infection. Although Heidi is familiar with the idea, she can't speak to its efficacy. Heidi promises the patient that she and Dr. Joanna will look into the procedure and get back to her with more clinical information at her next visit.

Dr. Joanna and Heidi understand that C. Diff is greatly affecting the life of their patient. Their first step involves writing a PICOT question. They work together to form the following PICOT question:

In patients with irritable bowel syndrome who suffer from recurrent C. Diff infections (P), how does the use of fecal transplantation (I) compared to antibiotic treatment (C) affect permanent C. Diff infection resolution (O) after transplantation (T)?

Dr. Joanna and Heidi discuss the terms they will use to keyword search each part of the PICOT question. Heidi jots down the terms they discuss, including fecal transplant, stool transplantation, antibiotic prophylaxis, and C. Diff infection. Heidi identifies the databases that she believes would likely have evidence to answer their PICOT question. She identifies MEDLINE,

CINAHL, and possibly Google Scholar as databases she needs to search. Dr. Joanna mentions that it would be good to explore whether there is a systematic review in the Cochrane Database of Systematic Reviews as well. While running the initial search, Heidi discovers two additional terms that she finds helpful—*fecal bacteriotherapy* and *fecal microbiota transplantation*—which she adds to the systematic search strategy.

Heidi finds several studies in MEDLINE and CINAHL that evaluate success rates for C. Diff treatment in individuals suffering from recurrent infections. In most of the studies, researchers found that fecal microbiota transplantation (FMT) had a fairly high success rate of 83–100%; however, researchers agree that the best route of administration is still a question to be answered. In discussing their patient's progress, Dr. Joanna and Heidi note that metronidazole is losing effectiveness in eradicating the C. Diff infection. This is particularly concerning given that metronidazole has been the first choice of drug for treating their patient's infection. Dr. Joanna suggests that she contact the researchers in the major studies in their body of evidence to see whether they have had similar situations. She also looks on the American College of Gastroenterology (ACG) website for any information that may be helpful. She finds a guideline that provides specific progression of treatment for patients experiencing metronidazole failure. She looks to see what evidence supports the recommendations. Dr. Joanna and Heidi discuss the recommendation for fecal transplant after three recurrences of C. Diff infection after vancomycin therapy. The ACG indicated the evidence was of moderate quality, and the recommendation was conditional (Surawicz et al., 2013). They discuss that there is no explanation within the guideline for what moderate-quality evidence means and conclude that they will discuss what they found with their patient at her next visit.

At the patient's next visit, Dr. Joanna and Heidi share the evidence they found, and informed discussion ensues about other drug therapies and the cost of FMT. Heidi is able to report that it has a low cost, with virtually no side effects. Heidi further informs her patient that because FMT does not involve drug therapy, there is no drug resistance, and the procedure has a relatively high success rate. After discussion with Dr. Joanna and Heidi, their

continues

continued

patient expresses that the "so-what" outcome is huge for her and that she would like to pursue this option for treating her recurrent C. Diff infections. She muses about how this treatment may help her get back to enjoying her former lifestyle. Dr. Joanna and Heidi discuss the patient's preferences with the internal medicine clinic's healthcare team. The team chooses to refer the patient to a gastroenterologist who performs the procedure, and an appointment is made.

Although FMT is not yet the standard of care, Dr. Joanna and Heidi feel that it should be offered to patients who are suffering from recurrent C. Diff infections and who have experienced treatment failure with traditional therapies. Heidi reflects on the impact of the EBP process that she and Dr. Joanna followed—the single question asked, the systematic search for an answer—and she marvels at how her evidence-based decision-making helped a patient dramatically improve her quality of life.

SUMMARY

In the past, searching for evidence has been somewhat of an "as you like it" activity. Often the steps and strategies for searching included searching the terms you wanted to and seeing what you found. The expectation was that whatever you found was the best you would get. Evidence-based practice calls for a systematic approach to searching multiple databases to ensure that the resulting evidence is relevant and can answer the clinical question. Systematically locating relevant evidence to guide nursing practice and improve patient care is an important skill that both registered nurses (RNs) and APNs need to master.

REFERENCES

American College of Chest Physicians. (2012). Prevention of VTE in nonsurgical patients: Antithrombotic therapy and prevention of thrombosis (9th ed). American College of Chest Physicians evidence-based clinical practice guidelines. Retrieved from http://journal.publications.chestnet.org/article.aspx?articleID=1159462

Eldredge, J. D., Hendrix, I. C., & Karcher, C. T. (2006). Core information literacy competencies in HSC curricula. Retrieved from https://repository.unm.edu/handle/1928/14373

Hartzell, T. A., Fineout-Overholt, E., Hofstetter, S., & Ponder, E. (2014). Finding relevant evidence to answer clinical questions. In B. M. Melnyk & E. Fineout-Overholt (Eds.), *Evidence-based practice in nursing & healthcare: A guide to best practice* (3rd ed.) (pp. 40–73). Philadelphia, PA: Wolters Kluwer.

Institute of Medicine (US) Roundtable on Evidence-Based Medicine. (2009). *Leadership commitments to improve value in healthcare: Finding common ground: Workshop summary.* Washington, DC: National Academies Press. Retrieved from http://www.ncbi.nlm.nih.gov/books/NBK52847/

Kim, S., Noveck, H., Galt, J., Hogshire, L., Willett, L., & O'Rourke, K. (2014). Searching for answers to clinical questions using Google versus evidence-based summary resources: A randomized controlled crossover study. *Academic Medicine, 89*(6), 940–943.

Melnyk, B. M., Gallagher-Ford, L., Long, L. E., & Fineout-Overholt, E. (2014). The establishment of evidence-based practice competencies for practicing registered nurses and advanced practice nurses in real-world clinical settings: Proficiencies to improve healthcare quality, reliability, patient outcomes, and costs. *Worldviews on Evidence-Based Nursing, 11*(1), 5–15. doi:10.1111/wvn.12021

National Clinical Guideline Centre for Acute and Chronic Conditions. (2015). Venous thromboembolism in adults admitted to hospital: Reducing the risk. Retrieved from http://www.nice.org.uk/guidance/CG92

Nourbakhsh, E., Nugent, R., Wang, H., Cevik, C., & Nugent, K. (2012). Medical literature searches: A comparison of PubMed and Google Scholar. *Health Information & Libraries Journal, 29*(3), 214–222.

Surawicz, C. M., Brandt, L. J., Binion, D. G., Ananthakrishnan, A. N., Curry, S. R., Gilligan, P. H., . . . Zuckerbraun, B. S. (February 2013). Guidelines for diagnosis, treatment, and prevention of clostridium difficile infections. Retrieved from http://gi.org/guideline/diagnosis-and-management-of-c-difficile-associated-diarrhea-and-colitis/

Technology Informatics Guiding Education Reform (TIGER). (2006). *Informatics competencies for every practicing nurse: Recommendations from the TIGER collaborative.* Retrieved from http://tigercompetencies.pbworks.com/f/TICC_Final.pdf

Younger, P. (2010). Using Google Scholar to conduct a literature search. *Nursing Standard, 24*(45), 40–46.

THE EVIDENCE-BASED PRACTICE COMPETENCIES RELATED TO CRITICAL APPRAISAL: RAPID CRITICAL APPRAISAL, EVALUATION, SYNTHESIS, AND RECOMMENDATIONS

Ellen Fineout-Overholt, PhD, RN, FNAP, FAAN;
Joanne Cleary-Holdforth, MSc, BSc, RGN, RM;
Pamela K. Lake, PhD, RN, AHN-BC; Tina L. Magers, PhD,
RN-BC; and Dónal O'Mathúna, PhD

KEY CONTENT IN THIS CHAPTER

- Identifying keeper studies through rapid critical appraisal (RCA)

- Evidence-based practice (EBP) competencies #5, #6, #7, and #15

- Evaluation of keeper studies from using an evaluation table

- Synthesizing relevant data from an evaluation table using synthesis tables

- Making recommendations from evidence synthesis

'Having gathered these facts, Watson, I smoked several pipes over them, trying to separate those which were crucial from others which were merely incidental.'

—Sherlock Holmes, The Crooked Man

SETTING THE STAGE

Rachael and her fellow operating room (OR) colleagues were discussing the recent spike in surgical site infections (SSI) during the last quarter. Rachael mentioned that she would like to find out what had contributed to the spike; she suspected that the new surgical residents were using povidone iodine (PVI) as a surgical prep instead of the usual prep of chlorhexidine gluconate with alcohol (CHGA). Her colleagues agreed that there may be an increased use of PVI in the OR cases in which new residents were involved in prepping the surgical patients (Step #0 of the EBP process). The group decided to formulate a PICOT question (Step #1 of the EBP process) to help them discern what the best practice approach should be:

In surgical patients (P), how does use of CHGA (I) compared to PVI (C) affect the SSI rate (O) post-operatively (T)?

Using the PICOT question keywords as their guide, the group gathered in the library to conduct a systematic search. They appropriately searched subject headings and saved their search to use later (Step #2 of the EBP process). They retrieved 30 abstracts to review and chose 15 for critical appraisal. Within the 15 studies, they identified two systematic reviews, one randomized controlled trial (RCT), one literature review with real-world application, five descriptive studies or EBP implementation projects, and four articles that they categorized as Expert Opinion (Level VII for intervention questions; see Table 5.1).

TABLE 5.1 LEVELS OF EVIDENCE FOR INTERVENTION QUESTIONS

Level of Evidence	Type of Evidence	Definition
I	Systematic review or meta-analysis	A synthesis of evidence from all relevant RCT and other studies.
II	Randomized controlled trial (RCT)	An experiment in which participants are randomized to a treatment group or control group.

III	Controlled trial without randomization	An experiment in which subjects are nonrandomly assigned to a treatment group or control group.
IV	Case-control or cohort study	Case-control study: a comparison of subjects with a condition (case) with those who don't have the condition (control) to determine characteristics that might predict the condition. Cohort study: observation of a group(s) called a cohort(s) to determine the development of an outcome(s), such as a disease.
V	Systematic review of qualitative or descriptive studies	A synthesis of evidence from qualitative or descriptive studies to answer a clinical question.
VI	Qualitative or descriptive study	Qualitative study: data gathered through interviews and other in-depth explorations to understand experiences and phenomena: the why and how decisions are made. Descriptive study: provides background information on what, where, and when of a topic of interest.
VII	Opinion or consensus	Authoritative opinion of an expert or expert committee.

Source: Adapted from Melnyk & Fineout-Overholt (2015)

The group consulted with their unit-based EBP mentor and determined that they needed the following RCA checklists to appraise the studies: systematic review, meta-analysis, RCT, descriptive studies, and EBP implementation projects. Their EBP mentor had access to these checklists from a prior project she had completed. She encouraged the group that they were effectively engaging evidence-based decision-making (EBDM), which could make an important difference in patient outcomes. After conducting RCA of the 15 studies, they determined that only three were keeper studies because their methods were done well and relevant to the question.

The final yield to guide the group's work was a meta-analysis (Noorani, Rabeys, Walsh, & Davies, 2010), an RCT (Darouiche et al., 2010), and a real-world translation of evidence into practice (Poulin, Chapman, McGahan, Austen, &

Schuler, 2014). The group, led by the EBP mentor, began to extract data from each of these three articles to place in an evaluation table. As the data were entered into the evaluation table, the group began to see commonalities across the evidence. They created a levels-of-evidence (LOE) synthesis table to readily show the rest of the OR staff the body of evidence at a glance.

As they talked about the evidence, it became clear to the group that the study findings demonstrated that alcohol may have made the difference in the SSI rate given that CHGA had alcohol and PVI did not. There were no studies that compared PVI with alcohol with CHGA; therefore, the group created a synthesis table that described the impact of the interventions (i.e., CHGA and PVI) on the outcome (i.e., SSI). As the group pondered the outcome synthesis table, they determined that their recommendation would be that all clinicians use CHGA for surgical prep unless it was contraindicated (Step #4 of the EBP process).

The EBP mentor discussed with Rachael about how she wanted to bring the information to the entire OR. They found a surgeon champion who partnered with them to draft a policy and an implementation protocol plan. The nurse manager provided her input regarding providing inservice education for the staff, residents, and surgeons on the new policy. Surgical site infections, which were monitored for 1 month after the protocol launched, dropped to below the national average (Step #5 of the EBP process). Given that Rachael, her EBP mentor, and OR colleagues were in a small regional facility of a large healthcare system, the group wrote a report on their work, including the drop in SSI, and submitted it to the system-wide Quality Council. The Quality Council discussed with Rachael and her colleagues about how they would recommend integrating the policy and its supporting evidence into resident orientation as well as OR orientation. After the policy had been in place system-wide and regular monitoring of outcomes was established, the group submitted an abstract to present their work at the annual conference for the Association of periOperative Registered Nurses (AORN) (Step #6 of the EBP process).

Whether it is healthcare or what is being purchased for dinner tonight, how we make decisions is key to achieving best "so-what" outcomes. Nurses have made great strides since the days of Florence Nightingale and the perception that we are handmaidens of other healthcare providers. Evidence-based clinical decision-making is the key to interprofessional practice, in which the primary focus of members of the healthcare team is on maximizing patient outcomes. To remove political wrangling and other sticky wickets from the conversation, the work we do must remain focused on the patient. Understanding how to appraise what we already know from research is an essential skill. It levels the decision-making playing field and refocuses efforts toward what is ultimately why healthcare exists: to help patients achieve optimal health.

This chapter discusses EBP competencies focused on critical appraisal, Step #4 of the EBP process. First, we explore the term *appraisal*. Often, *critique* is used to describe the evaluation of research or other sources of evidence; however, critique has come to have a negative connotation: finding the flaws in existing research. In appraisal, the focus is on the worth of the evidence to clinical decision-making. It is imperative that clinicians and researchers can and do critically appraise research. If the end result of research is its worth to practice (i.e., EBDM), then how we conduct the research and how we use it may converge.

UNDERSTANDING THE CRITICAL APPRAISAL PROCESS

Several major concepts within the appraisal of external evidence (i.e., research) are important to discuss. One is the leveling of evidence. *Leveling systems* parse research evidence into different hierarchical categories that are designed to help clinicians discern the relevance of different types of studies to different practice questions, with the caveat that the research is well done. Leveling systems have evolved with a focus on EBDM; several systems are available. Systems like that in Table 5.1 offer basic leveling of research designs to answer a particular type of clinical question: intervention questions. It is important to recognize that one single leveling system does not address all clinical questions; rather, different leveling systems address which research designs offer the best available evidence for answering different types of clinical questions.

Organizations have further developed leveling systems to meet their needs, such as the GRADE leveling system used by the Agency for Healthcare Research and Quality and many other organizations (AHRQ, 2013). The GRADE system was developed to offer a standardized approach to rating evidence (http://www. gradeworkinggroup.org/).

Critical appraisal uses levels of evidence to guide the thinking about what is known. The higher the level of evidence (i.e., mostly high-level research designs, such as RCTs or systematic reviews for intervention questions), the more confident you can be that the intervention will bring about the outcome you expect. However, without lower levels of evidence to help understand how the intervention works, the full benefit of the intervention cannot be realized. Therefore, the whole body of evidence must be included in the appraisal—that is, include all the information that is available to answer the clinical question.

Do not be confused by the different leveling systems for the same type of PICOT question (e.g., intervention questions) because most are complementary and serve clinicians well to advance practice.

Evidence-based decision making has a limiting factor. You cannot have confidence in *what* you do or *how* you do it unless you have evidence that reliably informs you about the effectiveness of what to do and quality of how to do it (i.e., valid and reliable research). Appraisal allows you to discern which of the available studies are relevant, valid, reliable, and applicable evidence for the current clinical question. Evidence that meets the appraisal criteria for establishing relevance, validity, reliability, and applicability goes into the body of evidence for making decisions; evidence that is appraised as not meeting these criteria (e.g., poor research methodology, inappropriate research design, inapplicable population) is rejected. Consider that a body of evidence is not defined by just a few studies but instead all that you can find about a topic: hence, the idea of "all we know" about a clinical issue.

Here are the four parts to the entire process of critical appraisal:

- Rapid critical appraisal

- Evaluation

- Synthesis

- Recommendations

Rapid Critical Appraisal

Rapid critical appraisal, as the starting point, is designed to discern what studies are retained as part of the body of evidence to answer a clinical question. Within RCA, three concepts are addressed:

- **Validity:** Did the researchers do a good job of conducting their research?

- **Reliability:** Do the findings indicate that clinicians can also get close to what the researchers found in the study?

- **Applicability:** Is the study appropriate to use with my population of patients?

For every study, some basics about the study need to be explored before gathering the data about validity, reliability, and applicability. This is the general appraisal overview (GAO). See Figure 5.1 for the GAO form template. Appendix B contains an example of a completed GAO form.

After the GAO is completed, the RCA process continues with evaluation of the three main concepts (validity, reliability, applicability) and how the article meets criteria for each concept. You would choose an RCA that is appropriate for the research design of the study you are evaluating. If it is pre-appraised evidence, such as a systematic review, meta-analysis, or guideline, you would use the RCA checklists for those designs. There are RCA checklists for most research designs, and they can be obtained by contacting the primary chapter author. Figure 5.2 shows an RCA checklist for RCTs. Appendix C contains an example of a completed RCA checklist for RCTs.

General Appraisal Overview for All Study Designs
Date: **Reviewer(s) name(s):**
Article citation (APA):
PICOT Question: *TIP: The PICOT question is not developed from the article. It is the clinical question you are trying to answer with the body of evidence.*
Overview of Study
Purpose of study: *TIP: Most of the information for the GAO can be found in the abstract.*
Study Design: *TIP: Include the study design and the level of evidence for the type of clinical question asked.*
Ethics Review Demonstrated (IRB noted): *TIP: Putting page numbers where information is located is helpful should you need to go back to the study for any reason.*
General Description of Study: *TIP: Include why the study is being conducted and what is expected to be accomplished.*
Research question(s) or hypotheses: *TIP: Hypotheses are statements that are made based on prior research and theory that provide guidance about what might occur within the study; Research questions are questions because there is not enough prior research or theory to guide the study. Research questions are exploratory.*
Study aims: *TIP: Sometimes purpose and aims can be similar – there is no worry to repeat, if indeed they are the same. Often though, the aim may be more specific than the purpose. Be careful to think about them individually.*
Sampling Technique, Sample Size & Characteristics: *TIP: Include specifics about how the sample was obtained, how many were in the sample and if these are appropriate for the study design. Provide information about the sample so that there is a clear understanding of who is in the study.*
Major variables studied: *TIP: Include the independent variable (IV) and the dependent (outcome) variable(s) (DV). Include their definitions and how the DV is measured.*
Statistical Analysis (include whether appropriate to answer research questions/hypothesis): *TIP: Only include statistics that demonstrate outcomes of the PICOT question. Leave all other statistics off.*
Conclusions: *TIP: Include the author's conclusion as well as your own conclusion for the study.*
NOTES for using GAO: This form is a working form that enables clinicians to document their thinking about a particular study as they record factual information about the study. You may want to include Notes to self that indicate your thinking as you complete the form. Also there are **TIPS** provided that offer some words of wisdom for how to use the form.

Figure 5.1 A GAO form.

1. Are the results of the study valid?	YES	NO	UNKNOWN
A. Were the subjects randomly assigned to the experimental and control groups?			
B. Was random assignment concealed from the individuals who were first enrolling subjects into the study?			
C. Were the subjects and providers blind to the study group?			
D. Were reasons given to explain why subjects did not complete the study?			
E. Were the follow-up assessments conducted long enough to fully study the effects of the intervention?			
F. Were the subjects analyzed in the group to which they were randomly assigned?			
G. Was the control group appropriate?			
H. Were the instruments used to measure the outcomes valid and reliable?			
I. Were the subjects in each of the groups similar on demographic and baseline clinical variables?			
2. What are the results?			
A. How large is the intervention or treatment effect (NNT, NNH, effect size, level of significance)?			
B. How precise is the intervention or treatment effect? Note to self: The precision of the effect has to do with the confidence interval (CI).			
3. Will the results help me in caring for my patients?			
A. Were all clinically important outcomes measured?			
B. What are the risks and benefits of the treatment?			
C. Is the treatment feasible in my clinical setting?			
D. What are my patient's/family's values and expectations for the outcome that is trying to be prevented and the treatment itself?			
Bottom-line Conclusion:			
Form used with permission: Copyright, 2005 Fineout-Overholt & Melnyk. This form may be used for educational, practice change & research purposes without permission			

Figure 5.2   RCA checklist for RCTs.

It is important to keep in mind that meeting the criteria for one concept is not enough. For example, a study may have good methodology, but the findings may not be applicable to your population of patients; this would make the study inappropriate to include in a body of evidence. Evidence-based practice is a result of fusing together the best available external evidence, clinician expertise (including internal evidence), and patient preferences (Fineout-Overholt, 2014, 2015; O'Mathúna & Fineout-Overholt, 2015). Using external evidence is a skill that builds with time. The key question for clinicians to ask themselves is whether any of the information from the study that is compared with the key criteria for good research falls short enough to negate the use of the findings in practice. Those that pass the litmus test of RCA are keeper studies and are retained for the subsequent steps in critical appraisal.

Evaluation

The keeper studies move into the evaluation phase of appraisal, in which higher-level evidence is included along with lower-level evidence. Keeping *only* high-level evidence is not recommended because that approach does not provide a complete body of evidence (i.e., "all we know"). The question is whether the higher and lower levels of evidence agree.

During the evaluation phase, you create an evaluation table that contains essential components of the research studies (see Appendix D for an example of an evaluation table template). Information is prudently pulled out from the studies, put into the table, and then compared *across* all the studies rather than reporting information study by study. The purpose of the comparison is to find similar information across studies as well as identify common differences and gaps in the information. Be sure to explain in the legend of the table any abbreviations you choose to include.

Synthesis

The evaluation table allows you to begin synthesizing data from across studies using a method of extracting information into smaller, more focused tables called *synthesis tables*. For example, a synthesis table can be developed to display the LOE of all included studies (see Figure 5.3). Another common synthesis table that helps readers quickly view the gestalt of study findings is the intervention and outcome table (see Figure 5.4). Synthesis tables are the prevailing underpinnings of the final step in critical appraisal: recommendations. As you engage in the EBP process, it is important to note that synthesis is the power component of the process. The result of synthesis addresses the "so-what" question put to a body of evidence—does the body of evidence support current practice or does it guide recommendations for change in practice? Furthermore, the result of synthesis is what convinces stakeholders to listen to the evidence and support evidence-based change.

Evidence Level for Intervention Questions	Studies		
	1	2	3
Level I: Systematic review or meta-analysis	X		
Level II: Randomized controlled trial		X	
Level III: Controlled trial without randomization			
Level IV: Case-control or cohort study			
Level V: Systematic review of qualitative or descriptive studies			
Level VI: Qualitative or descriptive study			
Level VII: Expert opinion or consensus			X

Figure 5.3 Sample of level-of-evidence synthesis table.

OUTCOME: Surgical Site Infection Reduction			
Interventions	**Noorani*** Level I	**Darouiche** Level II	**Poulin** Level VII
CHGA	⬆ (6.1%)	⬆ (9.5%)	⬆ (9.5%/10.1%)
PVI	⬇ (9.8%)	⬇ (16.5%)	⬇ (16.1%)

Legend:

CHGA = Chlorhexidine with alcohol; PVI = Povidone Iodine; *= Higher level of evidence;

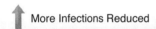 ⬆ More Infections Reduced   ⬇ Less Infections Reduced

Figure 5.4 Sample interventions and outcomes synthesis table.

Recommendations

Almost every research study includes a caveat at the end of the article that states further research is needed. This statement makes it challenging for clinicians to move to recommendations about the evidence. Conclusions such as "further research is needed" might lead clinicians to assume that the next step is more research rather than using what is already known in EBDM. Without moving to recommendations for practice, critical appraisal falls short of its aim to provide the best evidence for integration into practice. While more research may be needed, clinicians must make decisions based on the body of evidence currently available.

Consider that as you engage current evidence-based recommendations for practice, you must remember the potential for bias in both research studies and in the process of EBP. Bias may or may not make evidence unusable. The risk of bias from various sources should always be taken into consideration during critical appraisal (Higgins et al., 2011). Bias can be introduced as an inherent part of a study design due to funding influences, publication decisions, and other factors. When making recommendations for practice, the risk of bias must be acknowledged, but recommendations should be made, all the same.

TAKING A GROUP APPROACH TO CRITICAL APPRAISAL

Clinicians, educators, and researchers need to trust the EBP process, including critical appraisal, and follow it rigorously if practice decisions are going to be made on more than the opinions or preferences of healthcare providers. Healthcare needs well-done research, rigorously implemented evidence (EBP), and sound quality improvement to monitor ongoing outcomes. Nurses should be expected to seek out the resources necessary to make EBDM a lived experience within healthcare, beginning with the competencies listed herein.

Adhering to the steps of the EBP process should guide how these critical appraisal competencies are actualized in everyday work. Otherwise, these competencies could feel overwhelming. As you consider how to achieve the critical appraisal competencies, stick to the plan outlined here. Become familiar with the resources made available in this book and elsewhere (e.g., various table templates, RCA checklists). Visualize how you will engage the plan. Be sure to review the examples. Gather your like-minded colleagues to engage in meaningful group process, which can influence your ability to complete the work effectively. Learning can be accelerated through the group process, expediting the practice of critical appraisal procedures (see the sidebar). Finally, always keep in mind that practice helps critical appraisal (and other steps of the EBP process) to become easier and easier over time.

SAMPLE GROUP APPROACH TO CRITICAL APPRAISAL

After finding keeper studies, do the following:

1. Divide the collected evidence among the group.

2. Identify the resources that match the type of study you are appraising.

3. Report to the group the key elements of the resources.

4. Complete the resources (e.g., GAO sheet, RCA checklist) in dyads.

5. Dyads report to the group using their resources as a format for reporting.

6. The EBP mentor facilitates the process by prompting participants with relevant questions during the discussion.

7. A recorder fills in the evaluation table template as the dyads report on their studies.

8. After the evaluation table is complete, the group reviews the table for commonalities and gaps between studies and within studies (e.g., methodological issues) and discusses what they find.

9. A recorder fills in synthesis tables as the group discusses.

10. The group reviews the synthesis tables and makes recommendations for practice based on their review of the evidence.

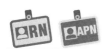

COMPETENCY #5

Participates in critical appraisal of pre-appraised evidence. (such as clinical practice guidelines, evidence-based policies and procedures, and evidence syntheses)

Strategies for Implementing Competency #5

- Learn the language (terms) associated with pre-appraised evidence:

  - External evidence

  - Internal evidence

  - Level of evidence

  - Pre-appraised resources, such as evidence summaries and synopses

- Develop knowledge of the various types of pre-appraised evidence that can inform clinical questions, such as systematic reviews, meta-analysis, meta-synthesis, clinical practice guidelines, EBP implementation and/or quality improvement projects, outcomes management reviews, or article synopses.

- Identify reliable sources for pre-appraised evidence, such as ACP Journal Club, BMJ Clinical Evidence, CINAHL, Cochrane Library, DynaMed, EMBASE, Essential Evidence Plus, *Evidence-Based Nursing*, Joanna Briggs Institute EBP Database, MEDLINE, National Guideline Clearinghouse, PIER, and UpToDate.

- Discuss how guidelines contain various clinical questions and their answers in the form of recommendations that are supported by a body of evidence.

- Learn how to determine the LOE of each type of pre-appraised evidence using a recommended hierarchy (rating system) of evidence.

- Gain skills in using general appraisal overviews, RCA for specific types of pre-appraised evidence, evaluation tables, and synthesis tables as part of a body of evidence.

- Choose the appropriate RCA checklist (determined by the type of pre-appraised evidence) to assess the quality of pre-appraised information and its relevance to EBDM.

- Make recommendations for practice, drawing on the conclusions reached from the pre-appraised evidence, to guide implementation of evidence-based patient care in practice.

Assessment of Competency #5

Is the RN or APN able to:

- Describe the scope and meaning of pre-appraised evidence.

- Use critical appraisal terms for pre-appraised evidence (i.e., language) appropriately.

- List the markers of well-done systematic reviews, meta-analyses, and meta-syntheses.

- Identify types of pre-appraised evidence, including systematic reviews, meta-analyses, and meta-syntheses; clinical practice guidelines; and evidence summaries and synopses.

- Discuss the appropriate level of evidence of the pre-appraised evidence using the hierarchy of evidence (rating system) that matches the type of clinical question asked.

- Use the appropriate critical appraisal tool (determined by the research design) to assess the quality of pre-appraised evidence (validity), its accuracy in patient care (reliability), and its relevance to clinical decision-making (applicability).

- Use pre-appraised evidence as part of a body of evidence for making decisions.

- Include pre-appraised evidence within evaluation and synthesis tables.

- Discuss how recommendations for best practice flow from well-developed synthesis tables that display selected aspects from pre-appraised evidence.

- Craft recommendations based on pre-appraised studies that are combined with other research studies in an evidence synthesis that leads to evidence-based decisions and best practice in patient care.

- Demonstrate use of critical appraisal of pre-appraised evidence in EBDM in annual performance appraisal.

- Participate in regularly held journal clubs that focus on critical appraisal: RCA to recommendation.

COMPETENCY #6

Participates in the critical appraisal of published research studies to determine their strength and applicability to clinical practice.

Strategies for Implementing Competency #6

- Determine the meaning of the phrase "critical appraisal."

- Learn the language (terms) associated with critical appraisal: for example, bias, validity, reliability, trustworthiness, and credibility.

- Develop knowledge of the various types of research designs that can answer clinical questions, such as randomized control trial, cohort study, case-control study, and qualitative studies, with such approaches as phenomenology, ethnography, or grounded theory.

- Learn how to determine the level of evidence of a research study using a recommended hierarchy (rating system) of evidence.

- Gain skills in using general appraisal overviews, RCA, evaluation tables, and synthesis tables as the tools of critical appraisal.

- Choose the appropriate RCA checklist (determined by the research design) to assess the quality of a research study and its relevance to EBDM.

- Learn to use evaluation tables to assist in evaluating across individual research studies.

- Learn to use synthesis tables to enable the display of common or disparate findings across a number of studies of interest for comparison and consideration.

- Make recommendations for practice, drawing on the conclusions reached from the synthesis of individual studies, to guide implementation of evidence-based patient care in practice.

Assessment of Competency #6

Is the RN or APN able to:

- Describe the scope and meaning of the phrase "critical appraisal."

- Use critical appraisal terms (language).

- Develop knowledge of the markers of a variety of well-done research designs, including randomized control trial; quasi-experimental studies; cohort study, case-control study, and qualitative studies; with such approaches as phenomenology, ethnography, or grounded theory.

- Determine the level of evidence of a research study using the appropriate rating system of evidence, based on the type of clinical question asked.

- Use the appropriate critical appraisal tool (determined by the research design) to assess the quality of a research study and its relevance to patient care decision-making.

- Discuss a body of evidence for decisions using evaluation tables with study data entered in a succinct manner for comparison and consideration.

- Discuss how recommendations for best practice flow from well-developed synthesis tables that display the findings from a number of studies of interest.

- Craft recommendations based on synthesis of research that lead to evidence-based decisions and best practice in patient care.

- Demonstrate use of critical appraisal in EBDM in annual performance appraisal.

- Participate in regularly held journal clubs that focus on critical appraisal: RCA to recommendation.

  - Using clinical scenarios, guide journal club discussion to markers of well-done research designs relevant to the scenario.

  - Determine the level of evidence of research studies using the appropriate rating system of evidence, based on the type of clinical question asked.

- Participate in grand rounds series (a meeting in which clinicians present health issues and solutions of a particular patient or population and invite the audience to participate) focusing on critical appraisal.

  - *Grand rounds 1:* RNs and APNs participate in using the critical appraisal tool that is appropriate for the research design being appraised.

  - *Grand rounds 2:* RNs and APNs participate in a team-based learning activity to put the studies into an evaluation table.

  - *Grand rounds 3:* RNs and APNs complete the critical appraisal process by providing well-developed synthesis tables from which they make recommendations for best practice to achieve patient care outcomes.

- Participate in an annual competency blitz. (A specified gathering of clinicians for the purpose of demonstrating competence in EBP skills through demonstration of the steps of the EBP process at designated stations.

Mechanisms for demonstration could include computer-assisted, such as searching, pen and paper, and simulation.)

- Successfully complete a quiz about critical appraisal terms (language), such as levels of evidence, body of evidence, validity, reliability, bias, trustworthiness, credibility, evaluation, synthesis, and best practice recommendations.

- Demonstrate EBDM at simulation stations that provide synthesis tables and require making recommendations.

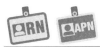

COMPETENCY #7

Participates in the evaluation and synthesis of a body of evidence gathered to determine its strength and applicability to clinical practice.

Strategies for Implementing Competency #7

- Determine the meaning of the terms "evaluation" and "synthesis" of evidence.

- Learn the language (terms) associated with evaluation and synthesis of a body of evidence: for example, strength of evidence, conceptual framework, abbreviations, legend, parsimony, bias, recommendation.

- Participate in choosing the appropriate RCA form (determined by the research design) to assess the quality of a research study and its relevance to EBDM.

- Participate in using resources/templates to evaluate each keeper study, such as RCA checklists (refer to Figure 5.2 for an RCA for randomized controlled trials) and *American Journal of Nursing* series, EBP Step-by-Step.

- Participate in using resources/templates for evaluation tables to enter all keeper studies' data to facilitate comparison across keeper studies (refer to Figure 5.3).

- Participate in identifying selected data in synthesis tables that effectively addresses the PICOT question, such as the effect of independent variables (interventions) on dependent variables (outcomes), levels of evidence, and study characteristics (e.g., sample size, setting).

- Participate in using resources/templates to create synthesis tables using selected data from evaluation tables of keeper studies (refer to Figure 5.4).

- Participate in suggesting practice recommendations from evidence synthesis.

Assessment of Competency #7

Is the RN or APN able to:

- Participate in a group to build an evaluation table from pre-appraised and single, primary studies.

- Participate in a group to identify in the keeper studies relevant data, such as:

  - Levels of evidence

  - Demographics of the study sample

  - Study designs

  - Independent and dependent variables

  - Analyses used to evaluate study data (e.g., statistics, content analysis)

  - Actual study findings (i.e., provide mean values in the experimental group and the comparison group as well as the p value or confidence interval, but do not provide a conclusion sentence, such as music therapy reduced oxygen consumption in the experimental group).

- Participate in a group to summarize the body of knowledge into two or three sentences.

- Participate in drafting practice change recommendations based on the synthesis of the evidence.

COMPETENCY #15

Critically appraises relevant pre-appraised evidence (i.e., clinical guidelines, summaries, synopses, syntheses of relevant external evidence) and primary studies, including evaluation and synthesis.

Strategies for Implementing Competency #15

- Explain the meaning of the terms "evaluation" and "synthesis" of evidence.

- Explain the language (terms) associated with evaluation and synthesis of a body of evidence: for example, strength of evidence, conceptual framework, abbreviations, legend, parsimony, bias, recommendation.

- Demonstrate the use of the appropriate RCA checklist (determined by the research design) to assess the quality of a research study and its relevance to EBDM. Include discussion of how bias influences decisions about the usefulness of studies to practice (e.g., some RCA questions may be answered as *no*, but there must be clinical reasoning to determine if that *no* makes the findings useless to practice).

- Use resources/templates to evaluate each keeper study, such as RCA checklists (refer to Figure 5.2) and *American Journal of Nursing* series, EBP Step-by-Step.

- Mentor RNs in gaining understanding of the concept that level of evidence plus quality of the evidence equals strength of the evidence.

- Use resources/templates for evaluation tables to enter all keeper studies' data to facilitate comparison across keeper studies (refer to Figure 5.3).

- Use resources/templates to create synthesis tables using selected data from evaluation table of keeper studies (refer to Figure 5.4).

- Identify selected data in synthesis tables that effectively addresses the PICOT question, such as the effect of independent variables (interventions) on dependent variables (outcomes), levels of evidence, and study characteristics (e.g., sample size, setting).

- Mentor RNs to use evaluation tables to assist in evaluating across individual research studies and pre-appraised evidence.

- Mentor RNs to use synthesis tables to enable the display of common or disparate findings across a number of studies of interest for comparison and consideration.

- Create and compile recommendations for practice, drawing on the conclusions reached from the synthesis of individual studies, to guide implementation of evidence-based patient care in practice.

Specifics for APN critical appraisal of pre-appraised evidence include:

- Identify resources that offer mechanisms to compare/contrast pre-appraised evidence housed within their websites (e.g., National Guideline Clearinghouse).

- Determine the credibility of the pre-appraised evidence.

  - Definitions for inclusion/exclusion of research

  - Look for bias, such as sources of funding, narrow perspective (vs. broad group of stakeholders)

  - Peer review

- Clear definitions of the leveling of the evidence to determine the strength of the evidence

- Use templates/tools to guide the RCA of pre-appraised evidence (RCA of Clinical Practice Guidelines; RCA of Systematic Reviews).

- Recognize that Clinical Practice Guidelines are a compilation of multiple recommendations. Each recommendation addresses a single PICOT question.

  - For recommendations that address the current PICOT question, evaluate the evidence base that supports the recommendation. Consider the grading/rating system used to establish whether the evidence base is strong.

  - If there is no rating system used to grade the evidence cited as supporting the recommendation, the APN will use templates/tools to guide the evaluation of cited primary studies.

  - If there is no evidence base provided to underpin the recommendation, the APN must mentor others in rejection of that recommendation.

  - With the current patient population in mind, consider the applicability of each recommendation (e.g., does the population in the studies match that to which the recommendation is being applied? Is the recommendation relevant to the clinical question? Is the recommendation feasible to implement in the current setting?).

Assessment of Competency #15

Is the APN able to:

- Lead a group to identify keeper studies through RCA, using appropriate resources.

- Lead a group to extract from the keeper studies relevant data, such as:

  - Levels of evidence

- Demographics of the study sample

- Study designs

- Independent and dependent variables

- Analyses used to evaluate study data (e.g., statistics, content analysis)

- Actual study findings (i.e., provide mean values in the experimental group and the comparison group as well as the p value or confidence interval, but do not provide a conclusion sentence, such as music therapy reduced oxygen consumption in the experimental group)?

- Lead a group to build an evaluation table from pre-appraised and single, primary studies.

- Lead a group to create relevant synthesis tables from selected data contained within the evaluation table.

- Lead a group to summarize the body of knowledge into two or three sentences.

- Lead a group in making practice change recommendations, including outcomes that indicate successful implementation, that are based on the synthesis of the evidence.

- Demonstrate use of critical appraisal in EBDM in annual performance appraisal.

- Lead regularly held journal clubs that focus on critical appraisal: RCA to recommendation.

- Lead grand rounds focusing on critical appraisal and use of evidence in practice.

- Lead in an annual competency blitz.

A REAL-WORLD EXAMPLE

MEETING COMPETENCIES #6, #7, AND #15

A group of pediatric nurses were discussing the most frequent complaint of their young patients, which was pain on insertion of an intravenous (IV) catheter to establish access for treatment and fluids. One of the nurses, Brandon, had been to a conference recently and heard a presentation on the routine use of intradermal lidocaine for IV insertion, particularly with pediatric patients. Brandon voiced his question in PICOT format:

In pediatric patients requiring an IV (P), how does routine use of intradermal lidocaine (I) compared to no lidocaine (C) affect patient satisfaction with the insertion experience (O1) and successful cannulation (O2) at time of IV insertion (T)?

The group was impressed that Brandon could rattle off a PICOT question so easily. He confessed that he had written many of them in nursing school. The group agreed it was a question that they would like to have answered. They asked the nurse manager whether she would support the project, and she agreed. She stated that she had been a pediatric nurse for more than 35 years, and pain on IV insertion had always been an issue for pediatric patients. The nurse manager agreed to pull one nurse out of the count for 4 hours per week to work on the project, with the caveat that if census or acuity demanded it, that nurse would have to go back into the count. The group made a schedule, week by week, for how they would accomplish the EBP process.

First, the group conducted a systematic search, which yielded 15 articles for further review. The APN met the group to help them start the critical appraisal of these 15 articles. She explained the importance of determining the worth of the studies to practice. The 15 studies were divided among the group members, and the APN made sure that each person had the appropriate RCA checklist to be able to determine whether his or her studies were worth keeping.

Each group member brought their reviewed studies and completed RCA checklists to the journal club meeting, usually held once per month. This month the journal club was held weekly. All 4 weeks were devoted to discussing the body of evidence to answer the PICOT question about intradermal lidocaine for IV insertion in pediatric patients. The concepts of bias and methodological rigor were discussed in the journal club prior to the group members reporting about their keeper studies and why they were deemed as such. At the end of the month-long journal club, 10 studies were kept to complete the critical appraisal process; two Level I studies—a systematic review and a meta-analysis—and eight Level II studies (RCTs).

With the body of evidence identified, the APN provided an evaluation table template for the group to use. The group members took turns entering their studies' data into the table. The APN would offer discussion points about what commonalities across studies were becoming apparent as the information was entered.

After all 10 studies' data were entered into the evaluation table, the group began the important work of synthesis using synthesis tables. They created three synthesis tables: levels of evidence, impact of intervention on outcomes, and definition and measurement of major variables. Across the RCTs, the study protocols were similar as well as the definition and measurement of study outcomes. The RCTs were congruent with the systematic reviews. Furthermore, the intradermal lidocaine decreased pain and increased satisfaction in the two Level I studies, as well as three of the Level II studies (i.e., RCTs), leading the group to come to the recommendation of routine use of intradermal lidocaine for all pediatric patients requiring an IV, unless it was contraindicated.

Steps were initiated to move the recommendation to standard of care. The process leading to this standard of care was presented by the APN and group at grand rounds, and a plan was announced for annual competency check-offs during competency blitz.

continues

continued

Pediatric nurses expressed gratitude for the synthesis tables that explained why the standard had been adopted. IV insertion forms now had a step in the procedure for intradermal lidocaine. The group reflected on their work and the impact they had made. They were pleased with the process; however, the real outcome was realized when their patients' parents thanked them for being so kind to offer a way for their children to avoid more hurt and to see the children sitting there smiling, IV inserted.

A REAL-WORLD EXAMPLE

MEETING COMPETENCIES #5 AND #15

Susan, the unit practice council chair, was collecting nurse-sensitive data for discussion at the meeting scheduled for next week. She noticed an increasing trend for central line–associated bloodstream infections (CLABSIs), and their data revealed the CLABSI rate was higher than the national benchmark for a medical-surgical unit. In the meeting the following week, the internal data of their CLABSI rate compared with the benchmark data were discussed. The nurses thought they were doing all the right things to prevent CLABSI, but they wanted to find the evidence to have confidence in their current nursing practices that were known to be effective and to discover additional interventions to their existing protocol for CLABSIs prevention to make them more effective. They realized that they were experiencing more complex patients with a higher acuity and multiple co-morbidities than ever before. Susan also reminded the group that hospital-acquired infections (HAIs) are an international challenge to healthcare providers and have been identified as events that should never happen by the Centers for Medicare and Medicaid Services (CMS) and, therefore, are not reimbursable costs. These HAIs are considered "never events" because the evidence is strong (reliable and valid) on how to prevent the infections. Keeping these details in mind, the council members paired up into small teams to search for the evidence. Susan and Erica said they would look for clinical practice guidelines, and they scheduled a time to meet in the computer lab.

Susan suggested they begin with the National Guideline Clearinghouse on the AHRQ website. They typed the keyword *clabsi*.

Their first priority was to scan the guideline looking for content that addressed their clinical issue. They knew from the EBP mentor at their hospital that they needed to evaluate all evidence for validity and reliability. From the online guideline, they reviewed who had compiled them and were impressed that multiple experts from major agencies (e.g., IDSA, CDC, SHEA) in the field of infection prevention had participated in the collection, evaluation, and synthesis of the evidence. It was published by the Centers for Disease Control and Prevention (CDC) in 2011. The lists of interventions were categorized in an easy to understand format and provided the strength of the evidence for each of the recommendations based on the GRADE rating system by AHRQ.

Overall, Susan and Erica thought this guideline would be helpful to their council and completed the appropriate RCA tool to make sure they had not missed anything before deciding to use the guideline as their evidence for validating and enhancing their existing practice. Erica suggested that they look for other guidelines from some of the national agencies on infection prevention. Although the CDC guideline was published in 2011, Erica wondered about newer information published by other organizations. Susan agreed, and they looked at the Association for Professionals in Infection Control (APIC) and Joint Commission websites for more guidelines, but they did not find any newer information.

Before they reported back to the team, they pulled information from the guideline with its supportive evidence to make the evidence base very clear to the staff. They used an evaluation table to pull elements of the guideline recommendations and the grade of the evidentiary support. In a synthesis table, they documented the commonalities between the guideline recommendations with the highest levels of evidence and their current practices. There were so many recommendations within this one guideline, and they wanted to make sure they didn't miss any new practices that could add to

continues

continued

> their bundle of care for patients with a central vascular device. They found two recommendations that were inconsistently followed in practice. Heightened awareness among the nurses resulted in a reduction in CLABSI in the following quarter. The group was pleased with the initiation and follow-through in using pre-appraised evidence to validate and improve their care and subsequent outcomes.

SUMMARY

Critical appraisal of evidence is the heart of the EBP process. Everything before in the EBP process flows into critical appraisal, and everything after flows out of it. Critical appraisal is multifaceted and likely will require some time and effort to demonstrate competence. Therefore, only the best evidence, that which is valid, reliable, and applicable, becomes part of the evidence-based decision. Patients deserve to have clinicians who are caring for them make the best decisions that are based on the best knowledge. Competence in critical appraisal is key to achieving best outcomes.

REFERENCES

Agency for Healthcare Research and Quality (AHRQ). (2013). Methods guide for comparative effectiveness reviews. Grading the strength of a body of evidence when assessing health care interventions for the effective health care program of the Agency for Healthcare Research and Quality: An update. Retrieved from http://www.effectivehealthcare.ahrq.gov/ehc/products/457/1752/methods-guidance-grading-evidence-131118.pdf

Darouiche, R. O., Wall, M. J., Itani, K., Otterson, M., Webb, A. L., Carrick, M. M., . . . Berger, D. H. (2010). Chlorhexidine-alcohol versus povidone-iodine for surgical-site antisepsis. *New England Journal of Medicine, 362*, 18–26. doi:10.1056/NEJMoa0810988

Fineout-Overholt, E. (2014). EBP, QI & research: Kindred spirits or strange bedfellows. In C. B. Hedges & B. Williams, *Anatomy of research for nurses: A practical approach*. Indianapolis, IN: Sigma Theta Tau International.

Fineout-Overholt, E. (2015). Getting best outcomes: Paradigm and process matter. *Worldviews on Evidence-Based Nursing, 12*(4), 183–186.

Higgins, J. P. T., Altman, D. G., Gøtzsche, P. C., Jüni, P., Moher, D., Oxman, A. D., ... Savovi, J. (2011). The Cochrane Collaboration's tool for assessing risk of bias in randomised trials. *BMJ, 343*, 1–9. doi:http://dx.doi.org/10.1136/bmj.d5928

Melnyk, B. M., & Fineout-Overholt, E. (2015). *Evidence-based practice in nursing and healthcare: A guide to best practice* (3rd ed.). Philadelphia, PA: Lippincott, Williams & Wilkins.

Noorani, A., Rabeys, N., Walsh, S. R., & Davies, R. J. (2010). Systematic review and meta-analysis of preoperative antisepsis with chlorhexidine versus povidone–iodine in clean-contaminated surgery. *British Journal of Surgery, 97*, 1614–1620.

O'Mathúna, D. P., & Fineout-Overholt, E. (2015). Critically appraising quantitative evidence for clinical decision-making. In B. M. Melnyk & E. Fineout-Overholt, *Evidence-based practice in nursing and healthcare: A guide to best practice* (3rd ed.) (pp. 81–134). Philadelphia, PA: Wolters Kluwer.

Poulin, P., Chapman, K., McGahan, L., Austen, L., & Schuler, T. (2014). Preoperative skin antiseptics for preventing surgical site infections: What to do? *Operating Room Nurses Association of Canada Journal, 32*(3), 12–29.

6

THE EVIDENCE-BASED PRACTICE COMPETENCIES RELATED TO IMPLEMENTATION

Lynn Gallagher-Ford, PhD, RN, DPFNAP, NE-BC

KEY CONTENT IN THIS CHAPTER

- Implementing an evidence-based practice (EBP) change: Planning for change

- Tools to guide the EBP change process

- Evidence-based competencies #9, #10, #16, #17, and #20

- Meeting the competencies for implementation of an EBP change

- Assessing the EBP competencies for implementation of an EBP change

- Real-world examples of implementing the EBP change competencies

SETTING THE STAGE

Maria is a staff nurse on a medical surgical unit in a large community hospital. She has worked on this unit for 7 years and has always wondered why the nurses are required to change IVs on their patients every 72 hours, even if the IV looks fine and is running well. When Maria questions her colleagues, her manager, and the quality director about this practice, she hears the following responses: "That is just how we do it here," "We've always changed IVs at 72 hours," "We change them like that to prevent infections," and "That's the policy." Maria wonders whether any research supports this practice (Step #0 in the EBP process) and contacts her unit-based educator (Nancy) to explore her question further. Nancy recently attended a 5-day EBP education program and is one of several EBP mentors in the hospital. Maria and Nancy meet the following day to discuss the clinical situation. Together, Nancy and Maria formulate the following searchable question by using a PICOT template (Step #1 of the EBP process):

In hospitalized adults (P), how does changing IV sites at 72 hours (I) compared to changing IV sites when clinically indicated (C) affect infection rates (O) during hospitalization (T)?

Based on the PICOT question, Nancy and Maria conduct an evidence search in the Cochrane Database of Systematic Reviews, MEDLINE, and Cumulative Index to Nursing and Allied Health Literature (CINAHL) and find 14 studies that look like they will be helpful in answering Maria's question (Step #2 in the EBP process). Nancy and Maria assemble a group of clinical colleagues who also are interested in finding the answer to this question, and engage them in a mentored journal club where they critically appraise the group of studies (the body of evidence) found in the literature search. With their EBP mentor's help, Maria and her colleagues synthesize the group of studies (the body of evidence) and come to the conclusions that (1) the evidence clearly reflects that changing IV sites every 72 or 96 hours is no more effective in reducing infection rates or the incidence of phlebitis when compared with changing the IV site when clinically indicated, and (2) that changing the IV site when clinically indicated was found to reduce costs compared with changing IV sites every 72 to 96 hours (Step #3 in the EBP process).

Based on the evidence, Maria, Nancy, and their colleagues make a recommendation to key stakeholders (infection control practitioners, medical executive chairperson, quality council representative, and the director for medical surgical nursing) that the IV policy should be changed to reflect the current best evidence: That is, IV sites should be changed when clinically indicated and not merely routinely at 72 hours. Upon review of the evidence, the key stakeholders agree that the policy should be changed, and each of them should take responsibility to present the evidence-based recommendation to their respective committees and then forward the recommendation on to the policy and procedure committee. After the policy is updated, their new evidence-based IV Site Management Policy and Procedure is rolled out to the entire organization (Step #4 in the EBP process). The infection control team and clinical practice council are assigned to track the IV infection rate data and phlebitis incidence rates, respectively, for 6 months after the rollout and report their findings to assure that implementation of the EBP change is having the expected positive effect on these key patient outcomes (Step #5 in the EBP process).

Maria and Nancy are pleased to see the data each month, reflecting that both of the key quality indicators are not just stable but are, in fact, improving with the new IV site change process. In addition to the positive patient outcomes, the nursing staff are excited about using their clinical judgement to assess patients' needs and intervening when indicated, not just because "that's the way we do it here." They also are happy to have more time to take care of patents' other needs because they are not spending time performing an unnecessary task. After 6 months, Nancy receives notification from the chief financial officer (CFO), in which he shares the fact that the hospital is tracking positive cost savings related to the new IV practice, which Nancy immediately shares with Maria, her nurse manager, and the nursing director.

Maria's manager encourages her to submit her EBP project and story to the regional research and EBP conference. Maria shares this idea with Nancy, and together they prepare and submit an abstract for a poster presentation that is accepted. Maria and her EBP mentor present their findings at the conference and win the Best EBP Poster Award (Step #6 in the EBP process). Maria's first EBP experience is very rewarding, and as a result, she joins the shared governance

EBP/Research Council where she is learning more about EBP and helping to lead the EBP culture shift in her organization.

IMPLEMENTING AN EVIDENCE-BASED PRACTICE CHANGE: PLANNING FOR CHANGE

Implementing an EBP change is the key point of Step #4 in the seven-step EBP process (Melnyk & Fineout-Overholt, 2015), which states:

> *Integrate the best evidence with one's clinical expertise and patient preferences and values in making a practice decision or change.*

This step includes all activities critical to preparing for and actually implementing an EBP decision or change. When an individual clinician is making an EBP decision, the process is relatively quick. A question is formulated; the evidence is attained, appraised, synthesized, and integrated into a decision; and the resulting behaviors/ actions implemented by the individual are evidence-based.

When an EBP change is being implemented on a larger scale (e.g., within a specialty unit, across an organization, or in a population practice setting), this step in the process is busy and potentially time-consuming because many individuals (stakeholders) tend to be involved in the change process. Change, of any kind, is not easy for many people, and managing change has been written about for decades. There are a variety of models and approaches for managing the change process that can be used when implementing evidence-based change (Rogers, Lewin, and Duck are three examples of models). Resistance to change is the behavior that is often exhibited during new initiatives, but the behavior of resistance is typically fueled by the emotion of fear.

Evidence-based change may be particularly challenging because individuals are uncertain and fearful of things they do not understand. So, when an EBP change is introduced, individuals who are experts at the previous "way we've done it here" may resist the change because they are fearful of being perceived as less expert, or uninformed, or even incompetent. These are very real and intense fears that are critical to understand and address in order to successfully change to an organizational evidence-based approach to decision-making and practice. With this in mind, it is critical for organizations to develop an evidence-based clinical environment that includes (Hockenberry, Brown, & Rogers, 2015):

- Creating a vision for EBP

- Promoting engagement in EBP

- Integrating EBP into the clinical environment

- Evaluating EBP in the clinical environment

It is critical to recognize that time and energy spent in creating a supportive EBP environment are invaluable investments in the success of implementing EBP projects and in ultimately living an evidence-based approach to all practice decisions.

When planning to implement an EBP change, expect many tasks and many human connections to be made. As the team that will plan and execute implementation of the EBP project, be sure to include individuals with a variety of strengths and interests. Some people are great at detail-oriented work, such as creating a project timeline or drafting a new protocol, whereas others are much better at the relationship building that will be necessary for the project's success, such as engaging key stakeholders or discussing potential barriers/facilitators with the staff who will be involved. Many tools are available that individuals can use to determine their personality and communication strengths. Using these tools to gain a better understanding of each of the team member's strengths is an excellent team-building activity, and the insights provided will serve the EBP project well and ultimately contribute to the development of a supportive EBP culture.

TOOLS TO GUIDE THE EBP CHANGE PROCESS

Every EBP practice change project should be planned and executed strategically. There are tools available to guide teams and provide structure to the process, including the EBP Project Planner (see Table 6.1). Note that steps in the process overlap and also this is a guide: Project timelines can vary.

TABLE 6.1 EBP PROJECT PLANNER

Project Steps	Estimated Time Frame	Notes
Identify the problem area/issue based on clinical inquiry.	1 week	
Gather and evaluate current practice data (collect internal evidence).	4 weeks	
Formulate a specific, searchable PICOT question.	1 week	
Identify key staff and stakeholders.	2 weeks	
Identify EBP project team.	2 weeks	
Conduct a literature search and identify keeper studies. Connect with the librarian (if available).	2 weeks	
Critically appraise and synthesize the evidence.	4–8 weeks	
Formulate the EBP change recommendation (or reach out to research colleagues when insufficient evidence exists to consider conducting a study).	2 weeks	
Develop an implementation plan and timeline with stakeholders.	4 weeks	
Recognize progress/celebrate success.	Ongoing, at regular intervals	
Identify outcomes to be measured. Include "so-what" outcome(s) in the plan.	2 weeks	

Develop a business plan for the practice change project, including projected expenses and return on investment (ROI).	2 weeks
Assess and address barriers.	2 weeks
Gain approvals (as needed).	4–8 weeks
Implement the EBP change.	2–4 weeks
Measure outcomes.	Ongoing
Analyze outcomes.	Ongoing
Present project outcomes internally.	4 weeks
Disseminate project outcomes externally.	Within 6 months after completion
Celebrate success.	Ongoing

Copyright Gallagher-Ford, Melnyk, & Fineout-Overholt (2015)

A project checklist, although not required, is a helpful tool to consider when implementing a practice change project. There are several critical steps to any practice change implementation plan including:

1. **Assemble a diverse and talented team.**

2. **Develop a timeline (and stick to it!).**

3. **Engage staff and key stakeholders in the process.**

4. **Provide information in a timely fashion. Make sure information is available 7 days a week and around the clock.**

   - *Visual:* Display poster/flyers about the project and timeline. Provide a location where people can write questions about the project.

   - *Auditory:* Create your *elevator speech* (a concise statement) about the project to enable conversations, answer questions, and create excitement about the project.

- *Tactile:* If using new equipment or tools related to the project, make them available for people to touch and establish a comfortable level.

5. Pilot the EBP change on a small scale when possible.

Starting small or with a pilot program allows your team to identify any glitches and correct them. A pilot also gives the staff involved an opportunity to ask questions, gain confidence, and develop a positive attitude toward the change before the larger scale implementation occurs.

6. Recognize great moments and celebrate success.

- Acknowledge early adopter/supporters of the EBP change.

- Provide recognition that reflects genuine gratitude.

- To accommodate personality types, provide recognition in both spontaneously and planned ways to both individuals and to groups in big (perhaps a party) and small (perhaps a personal note) ways.

- Recognize individual efforts/achievements.

- Recognize team efforts/achievements.

- Celebrate positive project outcomes.

Evidence-based practice changes require participation at every level in order to be successful. Practicing registered nurses (RNs) as well as advanced practice nurses (APNs) play critical roles in assuring the success of EBP in every type of clinical setting.

All nurses are expected to integrate both internal evidence (data from within a clinical practice setting) from sources such as electronic health records (EHRs), quality improvement or human resources departments, administration, clinical systems or generated through quality improvement, and outcomes management or EBP implementation projects (Melnyk & Fineout-Overholt, 2015) and external evidence along with their clinical expertise and patient preferences and values to plan and implement practice changes.

Advanced practice nurses are expected to support practicing nurses and lead transdisciplinary teams in gathering, understanding, synthesizing, and integrating the comprehensive body of evidence, from across varied disciplines, to inform practice changes to provide best care to individual patients and populations. This work is delivered in multiple ways including:

- Working with other clinicians individually to answer clinical questions

- Leading transdisciplinary teams to answer a clinical question

- Developing evidence-based policies and procedures to guide care for an organization

Because nurses represent the largest sector of the healthcare workforce, they have the greatest opportunity and potential to positively impact the transformation of healthcare from tradition-based to evidence-based.

COMPETENCY #9

Integrates evidence gathered from external and internal sources in order to plan evidence-based practice changes.

Strategies for Implementing Competency #9

- Identify sources of internal evidence within clinical units and the healthcare organization.

- Identify resources available to facilitate access to internal evidence (EHR, admission/discharge/transfer information).

- Identify human resources available to facilitate access to internal evidence (e.g., quality improvement specialists, professional development specialists, nurse managers, nurse educators, clinical nurse specialists and other APNs, other departmental managers).

- Identify sources of external evidence within clinical units and the healthcare organization (e.g., resources imbedded in the EHR, unit-based/intranet-based resources, librarian support).

- Identify human resources available to facilitate access to external evidence (e.g., EBP mentors, clinical nurse specialists and other APNs, nurse educators, organizational leaders, affiliated academic faculty).

- Seek out education related to gathering and appraising evidence (e.g., internal and external continuing education programs, college courses, EBP experts).

- Access EBP resources available and advocate for additional resources if needed.

- Practice EBP skills related to gathering, appraising, and integrating evidence (EBP mentor sessions, peer activities, journal clubs).

Assessment of Competency #9

Is the RN or APN able to:

- Define internal evidence and external evidence.

- Differentiate examples of internal evidence from external evidence.

- Describe how to access multiple sources of internal evidence within the organization.

- Describe how to access multiple sources of external evidence.

- Describe a variety of human resources within and outside the organization that are available to facilitate gathering, appraisal, and planning for integration of evidence.

- Access EBP mentor(s) within (or outside) the organization when needed.

- Demonstrate EBP skills related to gathering and appraising evidence.

- Describe clinical questions identified and the resources/processes used to gather, appraise, and synthesize evidence to answer clinical questions.

- Describe how recommendations for practice changes were derived from utilization of the EBP process.

 # COMPETENCY #10

Implements practice changes based on evidence and clinical expertise and patient preferences to improve care processes and patient outcomes.

Strategies for Implementing Competency #10

- Integrate the language of EBP in daily work and routine communications to promote understanding.

- Offer opportunities to learn about the relationships among evidence, clinical expertise, and patient preferences and values in making best decisions to improve care and outcomes.

- Use evidence in decision-making to improve care and outcomes.

- Encourage colleagues to implement evidence in decision-making to improve care and outcomes.

- Role-model implementation of evidence-based care in day-to-day practice with individual patients and families.

Assessment of Competency #10

Is the RN or APN able to:

- Describe the relationships among evidence, clinical expertise, and patient preferences and values in making best decisions to improve care and outcomes.

- Articulate EBP language accurately to promote understanding of EBP.

- Provide multiple examples of implementation of evidence into day-to-day practice with patients and families.

- Describe an episode of role-modeling implementation of evidence-based care in day-to-day practice to colleagues that promoted EBP.

- Identify opportunities to promote evidence-based practice change implementation on a unit and an organizational level.

COMPETENCY #16

Integrates a body of external evidence from nursing and related fields with internal evidence* in making decisions about patient care. (internal evidence*= evidence generated internally within a clinical setting, such as patient assessment data, outcomes management, and quality improvement data)

Strategies for Implementing Competency #16

- Identify opportunities to improve patient care and outcomes with an evidence-based approach.

- Effectively search for, appraise, and synthesize evidence from across disciplines to make recommendations for care to patients and populations.

- Publicly role-model integration of evidence into decision-making related to patient care whenever possible.

- Develop strategic relationships with key stakeholders and groups within the organization who are responsible for patient care decision-making.

- Effectively communicate the importance of integration of evidence into decision-making related to patient care with key stakeholders and groups within the organization.

- Influence key stakeholders and groups within the organization to integrate evidence into decision-making related to patient care.

Assessment of Competency #16

Is the APN able to:

- Provide an exemplar of:

    - The search for, appraisal of, and synthesis of evidence from across multiple disciplines related to a patient care issue

    - The recommendation(s) made, based on the body of internal and external evidence for care to patients and populations

    - The result of the recommendation(s) related to the specific patient care issue addressed

- Provide multiple examples of integration of internal and external evidence from across disciplines in decision-making about patient care in day-to-day practice with individual patients and families.

- Provide multiple examples of integration of internal and external evidence from across disciplines in decision-making about patient care in day-to-day practice with unique patient populations.

- Describe multiple examples of public role-modeling of integration of evidence into decision-making related to patient care.

- Describe interactions with key stakeholders where integration of internal and external evidence from across disciplines in decision-making about patient care was discussed.

- Describe interactions with key decision-making groups where integration of internal and external evidence from across disciplines about patient care was discussed.

- Provide examples of organizational patient care decisions that were based on integration of internal and external evidence directly related to his/her effective communication and/or strategic relationship-building activities.

COMPETENCY #17

Leads transdisciplinary teams in applying synthesized evidence to initiate clinical decisions and practice changes to improve the health of individuals, groups, and populations.

Strategies for Implementing Competency #17

- Advocate for the creation of evidence-based transdisciplinary teams as the standard for making decisions related to improving the health of individuals, groups, and populations.

- Develop transdisciplinary teams to address practice-related issues to improve the health of individuals, groups, and populations.

- Create the expectation of evidence-based decision-making from transdisciplinary teams making decisions related to issues to improve the health of individuals, groups, and populations.

- Provide EBP education to transdisciplinary team members.

- Establish advanced EBP knowledge and skills as a requirement for individuals leading transdisciplinary teams making decisions related to issues to improve the health of individuals, groups, and populations.

Assessment of Competency #17

Is the APN able to:

- Provide EBP education and support to transdisciplinary colleagues.

- Describe specific transdisciplinary team decisions related to improving the health of individuals, groups, and populations where synthesized evidence was applied and integrated.

- Role-model EBP knowledge and skills while working with transdisciplinary colleagues.

- Describe leadership activities that prompted/encouraged transdisciplinary colleagues and teams to apply synthesized evidence to initiate clinical decisions and practice changes to improve the health of individuals, groups, and populations.

- Describe leadership activities used when transdisciplinary colleagues and/or teams demonstrated resistance to applying synthesized evidence to clinical decisions or practice changes to improve the health of individuals, groups, and populations.

COMPETENCY #20

Formulates evidence-based policies and procedures.

Strategies for Implementing Competency #20

- Advocate for all policies and procedures to be developed by teams who are knowledgeable and skilled in the EBP process.

- Assemble teams who are knowledgeable and skilled in the EBP process to create all policies and procedures.

- Create the expectation of evidence-based decision-making to formulate all policies and procedures.

- Provide EBP education to policy and procedure team members.

- Establish advanced EBP knowledge and skills as a requirement for individuals leading policy and procedure development teams.

Assessment of Competency #20

Is the APN able to:

- Provide EBP education and support to individuals and teams who are developing evidence-based policies and/or procedures.

- Provide multiple examples of specific aspects of policies and/or procedures where synthesized evidence was applied and integrated.

- Role-model EBP knowledge and skills while working with colleagues and/or teams who are developing evidence-based policies and/or procedures.

- Describe leadership activities that prompted/encouraged colleagues and/or teams to apply synthesized evidence to develop a policy and/or procedure.

- Describe leadership activities used when colleagues and/or teams demonstrated resistance to applying synthesized evidence to develop a policy and/or procedure.

REAL-WORLD EXAMPLE

MEETING COMPETENCIES #9, #10, #16, #17, AND #20

Sue is an RN working in a cardiac step-down unit of a large university medical center. Recently, a patient on her unit fell while attempting to walk to the bathroom in the middle of the night and suffered a significant injury. The staff, as well as the patient's family, were devastated by this event, and both were passionate about working to prevent this from ever happening to another patient. The nurse manager asked for staff volunteers to help find out how the organization could do a better job of preventing falls (Step #0 of EBP) and to be on a committee to review and revise the fall prevention procedures on the unit. Sue volunteered to be on the committee, which was to be led by Marcia, the APN (clinical nurse specialist)/EBP mentor on the unit. The committee was made up of a mix of volunteer clinicians from a variety of disciplines, including nursing, pharmacy, physical therapy, and medicine.

The committee's work began with assembling unit data (internal evidence) related to falls that was provided by the unit's quality improvement council representative. In reviewing the unit's falls over the past 12 months, it was clear to see that the vast majority of falls were occurring:

- At night
- Between 12 a.m. (midnight) and 3 a.m.
- While patients attempted to use the bathroom
- In patients who were on diuretics

The committee decided to collect additional internal evidence by conducting informal interviews with patients who had fallen while in the hospital during the past 6 months. When they asked the patients what they thought was the reason for their fall, more than 75% stated that they fell while trying to get to the bathroom and that the fall was related to having to take their water pill so late at night while in the hospital. When the patients were

continues

continued

asked when they took their water pill at home, more than 80% stated that it was before dinner or never later than 5 p.m. When this data was reviewed, the team member from the pharmacy noted that diuretics were scheduled at 8 a.m. and 8 p.m. as the default administration times unless ordered otherwise. The committee members felt that the internal evidence was very interesting, informative, and compelling.

Meanwhile, the unit-based APN/EBP mentor was working with the team to formulate the best PICOT question (Step #1 in EBP) to help them with their search for external evidence to guide their practice change decision-making process. The team, with the guidance of the APN/EBP mentor, developed the following PICOT question:

In hospitalized adults (P), how does administration of diuretics after 4 p.m. (I) compared to administration of diuretics prior to 4 p.m. (C) affect fall rates (O) during hospitalization (T)?

The team did a comprehensive search in the Cochrane Library, MEDLINE, and CINAHL to find the best evidence to answer the question (Step #2 in EBP). They critically appraised and synthesized the external evidence (Step #3 in EBP) and concluded that many interventions can contribute to decreasing fall rates, including performing fall-risk assessments; performing intentional rounding/toileting; and targeted use of technology, such as bed alarms. They also found emerging external evidence that supported modifying diuretic administration times to earlier in the day if possible as an intervention that was effective in decreasing fall rates. The recommendation was that diuretics should be given no later than 4 p.m. or 5 p.m. whenever possible. In discussing the external evidence, the team verified that they were already doing all the evidence-based interventions recommended in the literature except the modified diuretic administration intervention.

Under the guidance and leadership of the APN/EBP mentor, the team created an evidence-based summary and recommendations and presented them to key stakeholders and leaders. When presenting the summary and recommendations, the team was strategic in selecting who would deliver the presentation to different groups. For instance, when the presentation was made to the Medical Executive Committee for approval, the physician member of the committee did the presentation along with the APN/EBP mentor. When the presentation was made to the Pharmacy and Therapeutics Committee for approval, the pharmacist member of the committee did the presentation along with the APN/EBP mentor.

After all the organizational approvals were received (with no major resistance), the internal and external evidence were integrated into a practice change (Step #4 of EBP) where the standard diuretic administration times were modified and no diuretics were administered after 4 p.m. unless there was a specific indication/order based on a particular patient's preferences or clinical situation. The new practice was piloted on Sue's unit, where there was a good amount of support from the nursing staff as well as transdisciplinary colleagues. The pilot was conducted to test the newly drafted, evidence-based policy and work through any glitches before rolling it out to the entire hospital.

The pilot went very smoothly; the staff was supportive of the change in practice to help prevent falls. Throughout the pilot, fall-related outcomes data continued to be collected (Step #5 of EBP) and were compared with fall rates prior to the practice change. The outcomes of the EBP project were very positive. During the 6 months of the pilot project, there were no falls at night (between 8 p.m. and 8 a.m.) on the unit. The effect of the practice change was very large, and the impact was a major improvement in the quality of patient care and outcomes.

The APN/EBP mentor, the nurse manager, and the physician member of the project team were constant champions for the project, and the team members did excellent work to integrate the best evidence into practice to improve patient care and outcomes. Individuals and the team as a whole were recognized throughout the project. Meaningful milestones were celebrated along the way with timely, genuine, and spontaneous recognition. In addition, major celebrations were organized related to the unit's sustained improvements at the end of the pilot as well as at the time of the successful organization-wide rollout.

continues

continued

Based on the pilot experience, no major changes were needed prior to organization-wide implementation of the EBP change to enhance fall prevention. The evidence-based policy/procedure was finalized and officially approved/implemented across the organization. Since the organization-wide rollout of modified diuretic administration times, the fall rates across the organization have significantly decreased, and the improvements have been sustained for almost 2 years.

SUMMARY

The implementation of an EBP project can be busy, time-consuming, and stressful. Projects generally involve many people and they require change to occur, which can be very challenging for some individuals to deal with. Careful and strategic planning along with utilization of tools such as frameworks, models, and planning checklists can help the EBP team and clinicians involved in the practice change succeed. Robust communication throughout the project and meaningful recognition along the way are critical implementation strategies to include in every EBP change project.

REFERENCES

Hockenberry, M., Brown, T., & Rodgers, C. (2015). Implementing evidence in clinical settings. In B. M. Melnyk & E. Fineout-Overholt, *Evidence-based practice in nursing & healthcare: A guide to best practice* (3rd ed.) (pp. 202–223). Philadelphia, PA: Wolters Kluwer.

Melnyk, B., Buck, J., & Gallagher-Ford, L. (2015). Transforming quality improvement into evidence-based quality improvement: A key solution to improve healthcare outcomes. *Worldviews on Evidence-Based Nursing, 12*(5), 251–252.

Melnyk, B., & Fineout-Overholt, E. (2015). *Evidence-based practice in nursing & healthcare: A guide to best practice* (3rd ed.). Philadelphia, PA: Wolters Kluwer.

Melnyk, B., Fineout-Overholt, E., Gallagher-Ford, L., & Kaplan, L. (2012). The state of evidence-based practice in US nurses: Critical implications for nurse leaders and educators. *Journal of Nursing Administration, 42*(9), 410–417.

THE EVIDENCE-BASED PRACTICE COMPETENCIES RELATED TO OUTCOMES EVALUATION

Bernadette Mazurek Melnyk, PhD, RN, CPNP/PMHNP, FAANP, FNAP, FAAN

KEY CONTENT IN THIS CHAPTER

- Defining outcome(s) and process measures

- Quality improvement/outcomes management

- Internal and external evidence

- Evidence-based practice competencies #8, #11, #15, #18, #19, and #21

- Meeting outcomes evaluation competencies

- Assessing EBP competencies for outcomes evaluation

- Real-world examples of implementing outcomes evaluation competencies

> You have to be burning with an idea...If you're not passionate enough from the start, you'll never stick it out.
>
> –*Steve Jobs*

SETTING THE STAGE

Jordan is a clinical nurse specialist and evidence-based practice (EBP) mentor for a neonatal intensive care unit in a large children's hospital. She has noticed that the rehospitalization rate of her unit's premature infants exceeds 40%, which is distressing for parents and costly for her hospital. Jordan wonders whether there is a better evidence-based way to prepare parents for their infant's hospital discharge than the unit's current practice that might decrease the number of preterm rehospitalizations (Step #0 in the EBP process). She asks the following PICOT question (Step #1 in the EBP process):

In preterm infants hospitalized in the NICU (P), how does a comprehensive parent educational discharge program (I) compared to no comprehensive parent educational discharge program (C) affect rehospitalization rates (O) one month after hospital discharge (T)?

Jordan does a thorough literature search for the evidence to answer her PICOT question in the Cochrane Database of Systematic Reviews, MEDLINE, and Cumulative Index to Nursing and Allied Health Literature (CINAHL) (Step #2 in the EBP process). She critically appraises and synthesizes 12 studies from the evidence search (Step #3 in the EBP process). Based on the evidence found, Jordan decides to make an EBP change in her unit and begins to offer comprehensive discharge teaching to all parents (Step #4 in the EBP process). Six months after the EBP change is made, she accesses the data on rehospitalization rates of the preterm infants on her unit to find a 50% reduction in rehospitalization rates, which indicates a successful outcome (Step #5 in the EBP process). Jordan presents her EBP change project to the neonatal intensive care unit (NICU) nurses as well as at her hospital's grand rounds. She also submits an abstract to present her project at the upcoming Association of Women's Health, Obstetric and Neonatal Nurses' annual conference. Jordan is delighted to learn that her abstract was accepted for oral presentation (Step #6 in the EBP process).

EVALUATING OUTCOMES

Evaluating the outcome(s) of an EBP change is Step #5 in the seven-step EBP process (Melnyk & Fineout-Overholt, 2015). The evaluation of outcomes is important to determine the impact of treatments or practices and EBP implementation or quality-improvement (QI) projects on healthcare quality, patient outcomes, or costs (Melnyk, Morrison-Beedy, & Moore, 2012). For example, the outcome of placing a patient with hypertension on hydrochlorothiazide (HCTZ) might be a reduction in blood pressure (the outcome). As another example, placing ice on a sprained ankle immediately following the injury may lead to a reduction in swelling (the outcome). Monitoring outcomes is essential to determine whether certain practices or evidence-based changes are effective.

Defining Outcome(s) and Process Measures

Outcomes are the result of a healthcare intervention, treatment, or practice that can be quantified (e.g., number of complications, infection rate, length of stay in days). They can be measured objectively by observation or subjectively by self-report (Hockenberry, Brown, & Rodgers, 2014). For example, if you were to implement an evidence-based fall prevention program (the intervention) in your medical surgical unit, it would be important to assess the number of falls (the outcome) prior to implementing the program (a baseline) and also 12 months after implementing the program. If the average number of falls in your unit decreases from the baseline number, obviously the evidence-based fall prevention program was effective.

Differentiating process measures from outcomes is important. *Process measures* are those variables or factors that influence outcomes. For example, a nursing action process measure that may impact the rate of ventilator-associated pneumonia (VAP) (the outcome of care) might include how many times a patient is turned in 24 hours.

In today's healthcare system where emphasis is placed on delivering high-quality care at reduced costs, it is important to measure "so-what" outcomes (e.g., those that are important to the healthcare system) (Melnyk & Morrison-Beedy, 2012).

Examples of "so-what" outcomes include core performance metrics (e.g., infection rates, falls, catheter associated urinary tract infections), length of stay, complication rates, rehospitalizations, and costs. Because these types of metrics are now tied to reimbursement rates for healthcare systems, including them in EBP implementation, quality improvement, or outcomes management projects is important. If findings from intervention studies improve outcomes that are not important to the current healthcare system (e.g., patient uncertainty, caring), it is highly unlikely that the interventions will be adopted in the real world.

Quality Improvement/Outcomes Management

Many healthcare systems have QI or outcomes management (OM) programs or committees responsible for monitoring outcomes and making practice changes to improve them. *Quality improvement* comprises systematic and continuous actions that analyze existing data and lead to improvement in health services and the health outcomes of targeted patient groups (U.S. Department of Health and Human Services, 2011; Shirey et al., 2011). Although QI should be evidence-based, it is often conducted rapidly based on what individuals think may improve the problem (e.g., trial and error) instead of using the best evidence to make a decision about the change (Melnyk, Buck, & Gallagher-Ford, 2015):

Outcomes management includes a four-step process used by healthcare systems to define outcome targets, establish measurement methods, identify practices supported by evidence, and measure the impact associated with implementation of new interventions on healthcare quality (Brewer & Alexandrov, 2014):

- **Phase One:** The clinical problem is identified, outcomes to be measured are decided, and data sources for the outcomes are identified.

- **Phase Two:** The literature is reviewed and critically appraised to determine the best evidence to guide practice, and implementation decisions are made (e.g., how the practice change will be implemented).

- **Phase Three:** Clinicians are educated about the new practice, and implementation is carried out.

- **Phase Four:** The outcome data is collected and analyzed, and findings are disseminated to key stakeholders and clinicians. Additional opportunities for improvement also are identified.

Internal and External Evidence

Internal evidence is data housed within a clinical practice setting from sources such as electronic health records (EHRs), QI or human resources departments, administration, clinical systems or generated through QI, and outcomes management or EBP implementation projects (Melnyk & Fineout-Overholt, 2015). Internal evidence is not meant to be generalized to other practice settings across the country, but rather used for decisions about patient care in the setting in which it is produced. *Dashboards*—graphic displays often used to display internal data, such as length of stay, infection or readmission rates, and patient satisfaction—are helpful in assisting clinicians and administrators to monitor the impact of care being delivered. When existing data sources are not available to measure important outcomes of interest, it will be necessary to decide what measures and processes will be used to collect the needed data.

In contrast to internal evidence, *external evidence* is data generated from rigorous research, which is intended to be generalized to other clinical settings to inform or improve practice. The primary aim of PhD researchers is to generate external evidence by conducting rigorous research. Conversely, advanced practice nurses (APNs) with a Doctor of Nursing Practice (DNP) degree should be experts in EBP and the best translators of research evidence into clinical practice to improve healthcare quality and patient outcomes. Advanced practice nurses without a PhD can and should be part of transdisciplinary teams led by PhD researchers to generate external evidence to guide best practices. PhD- and DNP-prepared nurses should collaborate closely to reduce the long research-practice time gap to ultimately improve care and outcomes.

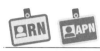

COMPETENCY #8

Collects practice data (e.g., individual patient data, quality improvement data) systematically as internal evidence for clinical decision-making in the care of individuals, groups, and populations.

Strategies for Implementing Competency #8

- Identify "so-what" outcomes that are important to the healthcare system to track over time for individuals, groups, and populations (e.g., core performance metrics, length of stay, rehospitalization rates).

- Determine best sources of the data and where it is housed.

- Meet with the "owner" of the data and inform him/her of your plans for an outcomes evaluation.

- Establish a plan for collecting the data and monitoring it.

- Integrate the data collected for individuals, groups, and populations to make the best clinical decisions about ongoing care.

Assessment of Competency #8

Is the RN or APN able to:

- Identify high-priority "so-what" outcomes for the healthcare system.

- Establish a plan for collecting and monitoring data.

- Use the data when making the best clinical decisions about care for individuals, groups, or populations.

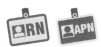

COMPETENCY #11

Evaluates outcomes of evidence-based decisions and practice changes for individuals, groups, and populations to determine best practices.

Strategies for Implementing Competency #11

- Approach other colleagues to determine whether a few of them might be interested in working with you to evaluate outcomes of an upcoming EBP change.

- Identify the "so-what" outcomes that are important to measure when an EBP change is planned.

- Determine where the outcome data is located in your organization and who owns the data (e.g., director of quality improvement) so that it can be collected and analyzed.

- Meet with the "owner of the data" to describe your outcomes evaluation project and data that is needed to evaluate the outcome(s).

- Decide on the time frame(s) that the outcome data will be collected.

- Collect and record the baseline data.

- Collect and record the outcome data.

- Use the data to determine whether the EBP change should be sustained or further refined for the continued improvement of outcomes.

Assessment of Competency #11

Is the RN or APN able to:

- Define the "so-what" outcomes of care that should be monitored for individuals, groups, and populations when an EBP change is planned or implemented.

- Describe where to obtain data to monitor the identified outcomes.

- Evaluate changes in outcomes that are the result of the delivery of care and EBP change.

COMPETENCY #18

Generates internal evidence through outcomes management and EBP implementation projects for the purpose of integrating best practices.

Strategies for Implementing Competency #18

- Identify a clinical problem with a "so-what" outcome that is important to the healthcare system.

- Formulate a PICOT question.

- Search for and collect the best evidence.

- Critically appraise the evidence.

- Integrate the best evidence with your clinical expertise and patient preferences and values to make a practice change.

- Evaluate the outcomes of the practice change.

Assessment of Competency #18

Is the APN able to:

- Consistently use the steps of EBP to improve healthcare quality and patient outcomes.

COMPETENCY #19

Measures processes and outcomes of evidence-based clinical decisions.

Strategies for Implementing Competency #19

- Identify process and outcome data that are important to measure when evidence-based clinical decisions are made.

- Determine where to obtain the data.

- Meet with the "owner" of the data to inform him/her of your plans for an outcomes evaluation project.

- Collect the data, track the data, and analyze it to determine effectiveness of practice changes.

Assessment of Competency #19

Is the APN able to:

- Describe process and outcome measures.

- Identify how the outcomes and processes will be measured.

- Monitor the processes and outcomes of care that is being delivered.

COMPETENCY #21

Participates in the generation of external evidence
with other healthcare professionals.

Strategies for Implementing Competency #21

- Identify important clinical problems that lend themselves to research, especially when external evidence does not exist to guide practice.

- Share identified clinical problems requiring study with researchers.

- Participate as a member of transdisciplinary research teams to study problems of clinical significance when opportunities exist.

Assessment of Competency #21

Is the APN able to:

- Identify problems of clinical significance that lend themselves to research.

- Share clinical problems requiring study with researchers.

- Participate as a member of transdisciplinary research teams to study problems of clinical significance when opportunities exist.

REAL-WORLD EXAMPLE

MEETING COMPETENCY #11

Hose is a registered nurse (RN) who has been working in the intensive care unit (ICU) of a 350-bed hospital in the San Francisco Bay area. He noted that the number of patients developing ventilator-associated pneumonia (VAP) has been increasing over the past several months and brought this concern to his nurse manager. Hose read a recently published article in *Worldviews on Evidence-Based Nursing* that investigated whether early ambulation of patients in the ICU reduced VAP. The findings from this clinical trial supported a substantial reduction of VAP with early ambulation, so Hose thought this might be a good practice to institute in his unit (Step #0 in the EBP process). The nurse manager agreed that this was a problem worth tackling and decided to create an EBP implementation team to address the problem. The team asked the following PICOT question (Step #1 in the EBP process):

In intubated patients (P), how does early ambulation (I) compared to delayed ambulation (C) impact prevalence of VAP (O) in the first seven days following intubation (T)?

A search for evidence to answer the PICOT question was conducted, and the studies yielded were critically appraised (Steps #2 and #3 in the EBP process), which supported that early ambulation substantially reduces VAP in ICU patients. Therefore, the team decided to change practice to implement early ambulation in their ICU (Step #4 in the EBP process). Hose volunteered to track the number of cases of VAP in his unit on a monthly basis and communicate the findings to the team. He approached the QI director in his institution about providing him this data on a monthly basis as it is gathered in the EHR system (Step #5 in the EBP process). After 6 months, he shared the data with the team that showed the number of cases had been reduced from an average of eight per month to two per month (Step #6 in the EBP process). The team concluded that early ambulation is effective in decreasing VAP with their patients and decided to sustain the practice in their unit.

REAL-WORLD EXAMPLE

MEETING COMPETENCIES #15, #18, #19, AND #21

Katherine is a cardiovascular clinical nurse specialist for a Midwest healthcare system comprising five hospitals. As part of her job description, she is charged with improving outcomes for congestive heart failure (CHF) patients. Katherine consistently questions the practices being implemented in her healthcare system, always asking whether they are the best practices to enhance outcomes in the patients (Step #0 in EBP). She has been monitoring 30-day rehospitalization rates for CHF patients who have had a hospital stay during the past 6 months and is alarmed that the prevalence rate has risen from 15% to 40%. Rehospitalization rate is a costly "so-what" outcome for her healthcare system given that it is no longer being reimbursed through Medicare. She begins to review charts of rehospitalized patients and begins to see a pattern in which patients who have not had comprehensive discharge teaching by their nurses (a process measure) have higher rehospitalization rates. She talks with and receives support from her nursing director to assemble a transdisciplinary team comprising nurses, cardiologists, and pharmacists to address the issue. The team asks the following PICOT question (Step #1 in the EBP process):

In hospitalized CHF patients (P), how does comprehensive discharge teaching by nurses (I) compared to other interventions (C) decrease rehospitalization rates (O) within 30 days of hospital discharge (T)?

The team did a comprehensive search in the Cochrane Database of Systematic Reviews, MEDLINE, and CINAHL to find the best evidence to answer the question (Step #2 in the EBP process). They critically analyzed and synthesized the evidence to conclude that comprehensive discharge teaching with CHF patients decreases 30-day rehospitalization rates (Step #3 in the EBP process). They also wondered whether a follow-up telephone call from a nurse in the week after discharge to assess how the patients are doing and whether they are following post-discharge instructions would also result in fewer rehospitalizations; however, the team found only one study conducted to evaluate post-discharge telephone calls, and it offered mixed findings.

Based upon the evidence from their search and combined with their clinical expertise and patients' preferences, they decided to implement an EBP change for all nurses to conduct comprehensive discharge teaching with CHF patients, including four topic areas: early signs and symptoms of CHF, how to monitor for a worsening condition, when to call their provider, and healthy lifestyle behaviors to optimize wellness (Step #4 in the EBP process). Katherine offered to take responsibility for accessing the EHR to track both the process (whether the teaching was conducted) and outcome (rehospitalization rate) of care with this CHF population (Step #5 in the EBP process) and will report the findings on a quarterly basis to the team (Step #6 in the EBP process). One of the cardiologists on the team also wants to conduct a research study to determine whether the comprehensive discharge teaching combined with a post-discharge telephone call would be even more effective at decreasing rehospitalization rates in this population than comprehensive discharge teaching alone. Katherine volunteers to be part of the research team that will conduct the study by educating the nurses who will be conducting the post-discharge telephone calls.

SUMMARY

Outcomes evaluation is a key step in the seven-step EBP process as it indicates whether the care being delivered is making a positive impact on patients, groups, or populations. When an EBP change is planned, it is critical to decide upon the "so-what" outcomes that will be monitored to determine the benefits, if any, of the change.

REFERENCES

Brewer, B. B., & Alexandrov, A. W. (2014). The role of outcomes and quality improvement in enhancing and evaluating practice changes. In B. M. Melnyk & E. Fineout-Overholt (Eds.), *Evidence-based practice in nursing & healthcare: A guide to best practice* (3rd ed.) (pp. 224–234). Philadelphia, PA: Wolters Kluwer.

Hockenberry, M. J., Brown, T. L., & Rodgers, C. C. (2014). Implementing evidence in clinical settings. In B. M. Melnyk & E. Fineout-Overholt (Eds.), *Evidence-based practice in nursing & healthcare: A guide to best practice* (3rd ed.) (pp. 202–223). Philadelphia, PA: Wolters Kluwer.

Melnyk, B. M., Buck, J., & Gallagher-Ford, L. (2015). Transforming quality improvement into evidence-based quality improvement: A key solution to improve healthcare outcomes. *Worldviews on Evidence-Based Nursing, 12*(5), 251–252.

Melnyk, B. M., & Fineout-Overholt, E. (2015). *Evidence-based practice in nursing & healthcare: A guide to best practice* (3rd ed.). Philadelphia, PA: Wolters Kluwer.

Melnyk, B. M., & Morrison-Beedy, D. (2012). Setting the stage for intervention research: The "so what," "what exists" and "what's next" factors. In B. M. Melnyk & D. Morrison-Beedy (Eds.), *Designing, conducting, analyzing and funding intervention research: A practical guide for success* (pp. 1–9). New York, NY: Springer Publishing Company.

Melnyk, B. M., Morrison-Beedy, D., & Moore, S. (2012). Nuts and bolts of designing intervention studies. In B. M. Melnyk & D. Morrison-Beedy (Eds.), *Designing, conducting, analyzing and funding intervention research: A practice guide for success* (pp. 37–63). New York, NY: Springer Publishing Company.

Shirey, M., Hauck, S., Embree, J., Kinner, T. Schaar, G., Phillips, L., & McCool, I. (2011). Showcasing differences between quality improvement, evidence-based practice, and research. *Journal of Continuing Education in Nursing, 42*(2), 57–68.

U.S. Department of Health and Human Services. (2011). *Quality improvement.* Washington, DC: U.S. Department of Health and Human Services, Health Resources and Services Administration.

8

THE EVIDENCE-BASED PRACTICE COMPETENCIES RELATED TO LEADING AND SUSTAINING EVIDENCE-BASED PRACTICE

Bernadette Mazurek Melnyk, PhD, RN, CPNP/PMHNP, FAANP, FNAP, FAAN

KEY CONTENT IN THIS CHAPTER

- Essential components of an evidence-based practice (EBP) culture and environment

- Attributes of leaders who lead and sustain EBP

- The ARCC model: A system-wide framework for implementing and sustaining EBP

- Evidence-based competencies #13, #22, and #23

- Strategies for leading and sustaining EBP

- Assessment of EBP competencies for leading and sustaining EBP

- A real-world example of implementing leading and sustaining EBP competencies

> "The greatest leader is not necessarily the one who does the greatest things. He is the one that gets the people to do the greatest things.
>
> –Ronald Reagan

SETTING THE STAGE

Kenan is a new chief nursing officer at a 110-bed rural community hospital in the southwest United States. He just completed his Doctor of Nursing Practice (DNP) degree and is eager to create a culture and environment that supports evidence-based practice (EBP) at his hospital. However, when he assesses the hospital's state of EBP, Kenan finds that many of the nurses and other clinicians have limited EBP knowledge and skills, and the culture is one of, "That is the way we do it here." Kenan wonders whether a continuing education course in EBP would strengthen his nurses' beliefs about EBP and enhance their implementation of best practices (Step #0 in the EBP process). He asks the following PICOT question (Step #1 in the EBP process):

In nurses working in rural community hospitals (P), how does providing an EBP continuing education course (I) in comparison to no course (C) affect their EBP beliefs and EBP implementation (O) six months after completion (T)?

Based on the PICOT question, Kenan conducts an evidence search in the Cochrane Database of Systematic Reviews, MEDLINE, and Cumulative Index to Nursing and Allied Health Literature (CINAHL) to find six studies that are helpful in answering his question (Step #2 in the EBP process). He critically appraises and synthesizes the studies to come to the conclusion that an EBP continuing education course of at least 24 hours increases nurses' EBP beliefs and EBP implementation (Step #3 in the EBP process). He develops a 24-hour continuing education program on EBP for his nurses that includes content found to be effective and implements a plan to have all his nurses complete it in 12 months (Step #4 in the EBP process). Kenan wants to evaluate the outcomes of the course, so he has the nurses complete two instruments (the EBP beliefs and EBP implementation scales) (Melnyk & Fineout-Overholt, 2003) before they take the course and also 6 months after completing it. In evaluating the outcomes (EBP beliefs and EBP implementation), Kenan is delighted to see substantial improvements in both (Step #5 in the EBP process) and presents his findings to his chief executive officer (CEO) and at the upcoming American Organization of Nurse Executives annual conference (Step #6 in the EBP process). Although the course improved the nurses' EBP beliefs and EBP implementation, Kenan is well aware that he must repeatedly communicate an exciting vision for EBP at his hospital and implement other evidence-based strategies to ensure a strong EBP culture and environment.

Even if clinicians are skilled in evidence-based decision-making and the seven-step EBP process, if they do not work in a culture and an environment (often referred to as *context*) where evidence is integrated into the structure of the organization to support them to deliver evidence-based care, their efforts are not likely sustained (Melnyk & Fineout-Overholt, 2015; Rycroft-Malone et al., 2013; Stetler, Ritchie, Rycroft-Malone, & Charns, 2014). For an organization to truly create an EBP culture and environment that sustains, EBP must be incorporated into the vision, mission, and goals of the organization and also made clearly visible across multiple venues (e.g., new employee orientations, visual displays throughout the healthcare system, the organization's strategic plan, clinical ladders, performance evaluations, policies, and evidence-based procedures) (Melnyk, 2014a).

ESSENTIAL COMPONENTS OF AN EVIDENCE-BASED PRACTICE CULTURE AND ENVIRONMENT

A key element of an EBP culture and environment is a spirit of inquiry where clinicians are consistently encouraged to ask questions about their practices. For example:

- In critically ill adult patients, how does oral care delivered every 4 hours compared to oral care delivered every 2 hours affect new occurrences of ventilator-associated pneumonia (VAP)?

- In parents of premature infants, how does light touch compared to rocking affect their infants' length of stay?

Without a spirit of inquiry, clinicians are vulnerable to falling into the trap of, "This is the way we have always done it," or, "This is the way that we do it here." With a spirit of inquiry, clinicians are motivated to search for the best evidence and integrate it with their clinical expertise and patient preferences/values to make the highest quality decisions about the care that they are delivering.

Evidence-based practice cultures and environments also contain the necessary infrastructure and tools that clinicians need to consistently implement and sustain evidence-based care, such as updated computers and access to electronic databases to enable searching for the best evidence to guide practice. In addition, these organizations have librarians who can assist clinicians in their evidence searches. Investments also are made in providing time for clinicians to implement EBP change projects, participate in EBP fellowship programs and continuing education offerings to further develop their knowledge and skills, and attend conferences to present their work.

Cultures and environments that support EBP typically have a robust EBP council comprising transdisciplinary clinicians throughout the organization who are passionate about and committed to the delivery of evidence-based care in interprofessional teams. Often, a director of EBP oversees the translation of research findings into practice to improve quality of care and patient outcomes. In addition, EBP is built into the job descriptions of advanced practice nurses (APNs) or certified baccalaureate nurses who are expected to facilitate evidence-based care throughout the organization. Healthcare systems that are steeped in EBP also typically have policies and procedures that are based on the best evidence and provide clinicians with evidence-based guidelines in electronic health records (EHRs) and through other mediums.

During new nurse orientations in strong cultures that support evidence-based care, clinicians are informed that EBP is an expectation for professional nursing practice. Further, EBP is described as the foundation for the delivery of quality healthcare, not something that is implemented on top of other nursing responsibilities. The EBP competencies for registered nurses (RNs) and APNs (Melnyk, Gallagher-Ford, Long, & Fineout-Overholt, 2014) are shared during orientation sessions with the expectation that all nurses and APNs meet these competencies. Including the EBP competencies in performance evaluations is a concrete way of reinforcing the expectation for the consistent delivery of evidence-based care.

Because of wide variation in EBP knowledge and skills of new nurses, organizations with strong EBP cultures invest in educational and skills-building sessions to ensure that their nurses and APNs are competent in EBP at the appropriate level. Dissemination of information alone is not enough; clinicians must be given opportunities to put their knowledge of EBP into practice to build skills necessary to deliver evidence-based care. An investment in EBP mentors—typically, APNs who are competent in EBP and knowledgeable in individual and organizational change—is important for advancing EBP in point-of-care nurses and assisting them with achieving the EBP competencies (Fineout-Overholt & Melnyk, 2015; Levin, Fineout-Overholt, Melnyk, Barnes, & Vetter, 2011). As part of their role, EBP mentors assess clinicians' competency in EBP and assist them in overcoming barriers to consistently deliver evidence-based care. Findings from studies have indicated that when EBP mentors are available in a healthcare system, clinicians' beliefs about the value of EBP and their ability to implement it increase (Melnyk, 2012). As a result, their implementation of EBP increases (Levin et al. 2011; Wallen et al., 2010). It also is important for EBP mentors to measure the "so-what" outcomes of their role, especially in terms of improving core performance metrics (e.g., complications, length of hospital stay) and cost outcomes (Melnyk, 2014b).

Attributes of Leaders Who Lead and Sustain EBP

Leadership competencies of chief nursing executives (CNEs) and chief nursing officers (CNOs) encompass the implementation and sustainability of evidence-based improvements in quality and costs, including creating structures to ensure access to information, resources, and support (American Organization of Nurse Executives, 2005; Everett & Sitterding, 2011). Leaders and managers who are successful in building and sustaining cultures and environments where EBP flourishes create a vision for EBP and communicate it clearly and regularly (Melnyk & Fineout-Overholt, 2015; Stetler et al., 2014). They not only support evidence-based care but also invest in a solid infrastructure that facilitates EBP in clinicians, including educational and skills-building sessions, time to plan, conducting and evaluating EBP change projects, having a critical mass of EBP mentors, and access to needed databases. They also "walk the talk" by role-modeling evidence-based decision-making. Findings from prior studies have indicated that role-modeling and valuing of research by nursing management increases the use of evidence in practice (Gifford, Davies, Edwards, Griffin, & Lybanon, 2007). Leaders' behaviors also are important factors in influencing staff nurse behaviors.

Research from a study of more than 1,000 nurses randomly sampled across the United States who were members of the American Nurses Association (ANA) revealed that the older the nurses, the less they desired to enhance their knowledge and skills in EBP (Melnyk, Fineout-Overholt, Gallagher-Ford, & Kaplan, 2012). This finding is particularly troubling given that the average age of a nurse in the United States is 44 years (Auerbach, Buerhaus, & Staiger, 2015), and most did not grow up with EBP. Further, these nurses identified that their biggest barriers to EBP were time, organizational culture, politics (e.g., "That is the way we do it here"), inadequate knowledge and skills, and nurse leaders and managers who resist EBP (Melnyk et al., 2012).

As a follow-up to this study that was funded by Elsevier, a survey was conducted with 276 CNEs and CNOs across the United States (Melnyk et al., 2016). The purpose of the CNE/CNO survey was to describe the EBP beliefs and implementation of CNEs/CNOs; their highest priorities; the level of investment in EBP; and their hospital's EBP culture, core performance, and National Database of Nursing Quality Indicators (NDNQI) metrics.

Findings indicated that although the CNEs/CNOs believed in the value of EBP, their own EBP implementation rate was low (Melnyk et al., 2016), which replicates findings from another national EBP survey with chief nurses (Sredl et al., 2010). Further, the highest two priorities of the chief nurses in this recent national survey were quality and safety, yet EBP was ranked at the bottom of the priorities, indicating a severe disconnect between the CNO/CNE's understanding that EBP is the direct pathway to healthcare quality and safety. Not surprisingly, 30% to 40% of the chief nurses' hospitals were ranked above benchmark on adverse outcomes, such as falls and pressure ulcers. However, it was surprising that the more than 50% of the chief nurses admitted to being uncertain about how to measure outcomes of healthcare services being delivered. In addition, nearly 60% of the

CNOs/CNEs believed that EBP was practiced in their organizations from *not at all* to *somewhat*. Further, 74% of the chief nurses invested 0% to 10% percent of their budgets in EBP (Melnyk et al., 2016).

This study has major implications for healthcare systems, including (Melnyk & Gallagher-Ford, 2014; Melnyk et al., 2016):

- CNEs/CNOs must acquire the knowledge and skills to role-model EBP and lead transformational change to cultures and environments in their organizations that support it in order to improve quality, safety, and cost reductions.

- Chief nurses must be taught how to present the business case to acquire more resources for EBP in their organization, including how to measure outcomes of EBP and its return on investment (ROI).

- Chief executives must invest more of their budgets to create and sustain an EBP environment if they expect their organizations to achieve the highest quality of care and best patient outcomes.

Changing culture and environment in an organization is a lengthy, often character-building, process that takes years given that there will always be people who resist change in an organization. Those resisters—often referred to as *laggards* in Rogers' Diffusion of Innovation Theory (2003)—are usually afraid of change. Open transparent discussions with clinicians who fear change can sometimes gain their support, but intense time should not be spent trying to convince resisters to join the culture change effort. A change to an EBP culture and environment can happen more quickly in an organization by getting those clinicians who are innovators and early adopters onboard with the change effort first and showing some fast successes by starting small and working on initiatives that can be more easily accomplished to demonstrate positive outcomes. An important question to ask clinicians is the following:

> *What is the smallest EBP change that you can make that will lead to the best positive outcomes for your patients?*—Bernadette Melnyk

In the words of Goethe, "Knowing is not enough; we must apply. Willing is not enough; we must do." Although building an EBP culture and environment is instrumental to stimulate and support behavior change in clinicians, persistent and consistent efforts throughout the journey will be worth it as evidenced by reductions in the lengthy research-practice time gap and ultimate improvements in healthcare quality, patient outcomes, and costs.

Studies on EBP have largely focused on barriers and facilitators of evidence-based care with clinicians. However, few experimental studies have focused on developing and testing effective interventions to facilitate evidence-based care. Further, there has been little research on EBP with nurse executives and their own practice of evidence-based decision-making. Studies that have been conducted with nurse executives have had similar findings to a recent U.S. survey (i.e., nurse leaders believe in the value of EBP, but their own implementation of EBP is low) (Sdrel et al., 2010). Therefore, nurse executives and managers must truly understand that EBP is a key strategy to improve healthcare quality and safety, role-model it themselves, invest in EBP educational and skills-building for their clinicians, and create an infrastructure to support and sustain evidence-based practice so that it becomes the social norm in terms of how all clinicians practice. Nurse leaders also must create an exciting vision and strategic direction for EBP that is clearly communicated, valued, and executed within the organization. They, themselves, must be the change agents for EBP and influence the way things are done consistent with EBP (Stetler et al., 2014).

As a follow-up to the recent national survey of 276 nurse executives, a national forum with more than 150 CNEs throughout the country was held in conjunction with a national conference of the American Organization of Nurse Executives. The purpose of this national forum was to share the findings from the recent survey and generate solutions to assist nurse executives with improving their own EBP skills along with determining the best resources and tools to help them build strong EBP cultures and environments within their own hospitals and healthcare systems (Melnyk et al., 2016).

The nursing executives at the national forum called for a bridging of the knowledge gap between EBP and healthcare quality and patient safety, as well as the need for educational offerings, specifically for them to enhance their own knowledge and skills in EBP and assist them in creating stronger cultures and environments for EBP. They emphasized that it is critical for nurse executives to be helped to understand the gap between EBP and its impact on clinical outcomes and return on investment (Melnyk et al., 2016).

THE ARCC MODEL: A SYSTEM-WIDE FRAMEWORK FOR IMPLEMENTING AND SUSTAINING EBP

Several EBP models exist, including the Iowa model (Titler et al., 2001) and the Johns Hopkins model (Dearholt & Dang, 2012). Many of the existing EBP models are process-oriented: That is, they outline sequential steps necessary for implementing EBP in a healthcare system. For example, the Iowa model describes a multiphase change process, which includes the following sequence (Dang et al., 2015):

1. Identify practice questions or triggers.

2. Form a team if the topic is a priority for the organization.

3. Assemble relevant research and related literature.

4. Critique and synthesize research for use in practice.

5. If there is a sufficient base, pilot the change in practice.

6. Institute the practice change if it is appropriate for adoption in practice.

7. Monitor and analyze structure, process, and outcome data.

8. Disseminate the results.

As another example, the Johns Hopkins model outlines 18 steps of the nursing process for EBP, from the practice question to the evidence to its translation into practice (Dearholt & Dang, 2012).

The Advancing Research and Clinical practice through close Collaboration (ARCC) model was originally developed as a framework to advance and sustain

EBP in healthcare systems (see Figure 8.1). In this framework, an organizational assessment is first conducted with three valid and reliable instruments (Melnyk, Fineout-Overholt, & Mays, 2008):

- The Organizational Culture and Readiness for System-Wide Integration of Evidence-based Practice Survey

- The Evidence-based Practice Beliefs Scale

- The Evidence-based Practice Implementation Scale

After the data from these three instruments are collected, an organization's strengths and limitations are identified, and plans to build on the strengths and overcome the limitations are devised and implemented. The key execution strategy in the ARCC model is the development of a critical mass of EBP mentors who are skilled in evidence-based care and knowledgeable about individual and organizational change. Changing organizational cultures and clinicians' behaviors from those steeped in tradition or the way it was learned years ago to one of evidence-based care takes time. Resistance is often encountered in the change journey as clinicians are often stressed by having to learn new skills or comfort with the way things have always been done. Evidence-based practice mentors have knowledge of Diffusion of Innovation Theory (Rogers, 2003), which emphasizes that it is important to first work with clinicians who are innovators and early adopters as part of culture change instead of focusing first on the late majority or laggards in order for an EBP culture shift to occur.

Implementation of the ARCC model deploys a critical mass of EBP mentors to work with clinicians at point of care to implement and sustain evidence-based care. When practice is facilitated by an EBP mentor, clinicians' beliefs about EBP rise, the level of EBP implementation increases, and healthcare outcomes improve. Multiple studies support the relationships in the ARCC model (Fineout-Overholt, Levin, & Melnyk, 2004/2005; Levin et al., 2011; Melnyk, Fineout-Overholt, Giggleman, & Cruz, 2010; Melnyk et al., 2008; Wallen et al., 2010). In addition, hundreds of EBP mentors are now working in healthcare systems across the globe to advance and sustain EBP.

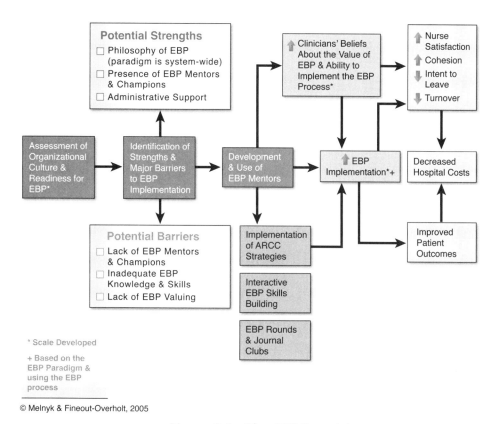

Potential Strengths
- [ ] Philosophy of EBP (paradigm is system-wide)
- [ ] Presence of EBP Mentors & Champions
- [ ] Administrative Support

Clinicians' Beliefs About the Value of EBP & Ability to Implement the EBP Process*

⬆ Nurse Satisfaction
⬆ Cohesion
⬇ Intent to Leave
⬇ Turnover

Assessment of Organizational Culture & Readiness for EBP*

Identification of Strengths & Major Barriers to EBP Implementation

Development & Use of EBP Mentors

⬆ EBP Implementation*+

Decreased Hospital Costs

Potential Barriers
- [ ] Lack of EBP Mentors & Champions
- [ ] Inadequate EBP Knowledge & Skills
- [ ] Lack of EBP Valuing

Implementation of ARCC Strategies

Improved Patient Outcomes

Interactive EBP Skills Building

EBP Rounds & Journal Clubs

* Scale Developed

+ Based on the EBP Paradigm & using the EBP process

© Melnyk & Fineout-Overholt, 2005

Figure 8.1   The ARCC model.

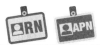

COMPETENCY #13

Participates in strategies to sustain an evidence-based practice culture.

Strategies for Implementing Competency #13

- Question practices routinely.

- Encourage colleagues to have a spirit of inquiry and to base their practices on the best evidence.

- Share best evidence/evidence-based guidelines with colleagues.

- Remain receptive to EBP mentoring.

- Seek opportunities to advance own knowledge and skills in the seven-step EBP process.

- Engage in EBP continuing education opportunities, EBP fellowship programs, EBP councils, journal clubs, and EBP or evidence-based quality-improvement (QI) projects.

- Participate in monitoring outcomes of EBP or evidence-based QI projects.

Assessment of Competency #13

Is the RN or APN able to:

- Question clinical practices on a regular basis.

- Encourage colleagues to question clinical practices and implement best evidence.

- Share best practices/evidence-based guidelines with colleagues.

- Demonstrate receptiveness to EBP mentoring.

- Participate in opportunities to advance EBP knowledge and skills, such as continuing education offerings, EBP fellowship programs, journal clubs, and EBP change or evidence-based quality improvement projects.

- Describe where to obtain data to monitor the identified outcomes.

- Participate in the evaluation of changes in outcomes that are the result of the delivery of care and EBP change.

COMPETENCY #22

Mentors others in evidence-based decision making
and the EBP process.

Strategies for Implementing Competency #22

- Assist clinicians with implementing the seven-step EBP process routinely in practice.

- Obtain knowledge and skills in individual and organizational change strategies.

- Develop ongoing skills as an EBP mentor.

- Assist clinicians in formulating clinical questions in PICOT format.

- Provide educational opportunities to assist clinicians in searching for, critically appraising, and synthesizing evidence.

- Assist clinicians in integrating best evidence with their expertise and patients' preferences and values in making evidence-based decisions.

- Assist the organization's policy and procedure committee with ensuring practices based on best evidence.

- Involve clinicians in EBP implementation and evidence-based quality improvement projects.

- Enhance clinicians' ability to evaluate outcomes of EBP changes.

- Provide opportunities for clinicians to participate in journal clubs, EBP rounds (forums where EBP change projects are presented), and EBP fellowship programs.

Assessment of Competency #22

Is the APN able to:

- Mentor others in the seven-step EBP process.

- Provide EBP continuing education/fellowship opportunities.

- Involve clinicians in EBP implementation and evidence-based quality improvement projects.

- Create teams that evaluate the outcomes of EBP change projects.

- Lead teams in EBP projects, including the evaluation of process measures and outcomes.

COMPETENCY #23

Implements strategies to sustain an EBP culture.

Strategies for Implementing Competency #23

- Gain skills in assessing the culture and readiness of the healthcare system for EBP.

- Obtain knowledge of EBP models that support and sustain EBP.

- Create an environment that facilitates a spirit of inquiry by point-of-care clinicians.

- Participate in the development of an infrastructure to support and sustain EBP.

- Advocate for resources necessary to strengthen the EBP culture.

- Formulate a strategic plan to sustain an EBP culture.

- Monitor outcomes of execution tactics.

- Role-model EBP.

- Recognize EBP accomplishments of clinicians routinely.

- Share outcomes and return on investment from EBP change projects with nursing leadership.

Assessment of Competency #23

Is the APN able to:

- Assess the culture and readiness of the healthcare system for EBP.

- Use an EBP model/framework to support strategies to enhance a culture of EBP.

- Facilitate a spirit of inquiry for EBP in the healthcare system.

- Work with leaders to develop an infrastructure that supports and sustains EBP.

- Develop a strategic plan with execution tactics to strengthen the EBP culture.

- Monitor outcomes of implementation strategies to support and sustain an EBP culture.

- Serve as a role model for EBP.

- Advocate for resources necessary to build and sustain an EBP culture.

- Share outcomes and return on investment from EBP change projects with nursing leadership.

REAL-WORLD EXAMPLE

MEETING COMPETENCIES #13, #22, AND #23

Latisha is a registered nurse who works on an adolescent unit in a 250-bed community hospital. She is troubled that she is seeing more teens hospitalized for medical conditions who also show signs of depression. Latisha is aware of the evidence-based recommendation of the United States Preventive Services Task Force (USPSTF) that advises screening for depression in teens in primary care settings when systems are in place to accurately screen for, identify, and treat them because she routinely accesses the USPSTF website for changes in recommendation statements. Although she does not work in a primary care setting, she believes that it would be beneficial to screen the teens admitted to her unit with the Patient Health Questionnaire (PHQ)-9 for adolescents, a valid and reliable screening tool in the public domain, so that those teens struggling with depression who are admitted to her unit could get an evaluation for depression while hospitalized with a referral as needed for evidence-based treatment when leaving the hospital (Step #0 in the EBP process).

Latisha takes her idea to John, a fellow staff nurse, who agrees it is a good idea to start screening the teens on their unit for depression. John and Latisha take the idea to their clinical nurse specialist, Jamie, who also functions in the role of an EBP mentor for their unit. Before taking the idea to their medical director, Jamie suggests that they should search first for evidence to determine whether screening for depression in hospitalized teens leads to better identification and referral for treatment. Jamie assists John and Latisha with formulating the following PICOT question (Step #1 in the EBP process):

In hospitalized adolescents (P), how does screening for depression (I) compared to not screening (C) affect the number of teens diagnosed with depression and referred for treatment (O) within a month after screening (T)?

Jamie mentors John and Latisha in how to search for and critically appraise the studies found in their search (Steps #2 and #3 in the EBP process). The best evidence supported screening adolescents on admission to the hospital, so Jamie, John, and Latisha took their evidence to the medical director of the adolescent unit. After seeing the data that they presented, the medical director and nursing team developed a new policy to screen all teens for depression when admitted to the unit (Step #4 in the EBP process).

Jamie assisted John and Latisha with developing an implementation plan to educate all nursing staff on their unit about the change and an evaluation plan so that evidence could be gathered about the impact of the new evidence-based change on their unit's outcomes. After 6 months, Jamie, John, and Latisha collected internal evidence on their unit to show that 24 teens who might have gone undiagnosed were diagnosed with depression and referred for evidence-based treatment upon hospital discharge (Step #5 in the EBP process). Jamie encouraged John and Latisha to present their EBP change project at the hospital's next EBP grand rounds and recognized their terrific work with an Innovations in EBP Award following their presentation (Step #6 in the EBP process). Jamie then offered John and Latisha an opportunity to participate in the hospital's EBP fellowship program, which she teaches. Latisha and John eagerly accept the invitation and look forward to enhancing their EBP knowledge skills and becoming one of their hospital's EBP Fellows.

SUMMARY

In order for EBP to sustain, it is necessary to create a culture and environment where clinicians are consistently supported to deliver evidence-based care. Evidence-based practice mentors as first described in the ARCC model are critical to implementing and sustaining an EBP culture and environment. In addition, nursing leaders must "walk the talk" and provide the necessary infrastructure and supports for EBP to flourish and sustain.

REFERENCES

American Organization of Nurse Executives. (2005). Guiding principles for future patient care delivery. Retrieved from http://www.aone.org/resources/PDFs/AONE_GP_Future_Patient_Care_Delivery_2010.pdf

Auerbach, D., Buerhaus, P. I., & Staiger, D. O. (2015). Will the RN workforce weather the retirement of the baby boomers? *Medical Care, 53*(10), 850–856.

Dang, D., Melnyk, B. M., Fineout-Overholt, E., Ciliska, D., DiCenso, A., Cullen, L., … Stevens, K. R. (2015). Models to guide implementation and sustainability of evidence-based practice. In B. M. Melnyk & E. Fineout-Overholt, *Evidence-based practice in nursing & healthcare: A guide to best practice* (3rd edition) (pp. 274-315). Philadelphia, PA: Wolters Kluwer.

Dearholt, S. L., & Dang, D. (2012). *Johns Hopkins nursing evidence-based practice model and guidelines* (2nd ed.). Indianapolis, IN: Sigma Theta Tau International.

Everett, L. Q., & Sitterding, M. C. (2011). Transformational leadership required to design and sustain evidence-based practice: A system exemplar. *Western Journal of Nursing Research, 33*(3), 398–426. doi:10.1177/0193945910383056

Fineout-Overholt, E., & Melnyk, B. M. (2015). ARCC evidence-based practice mentors: The key to sustaining evidence-based practice. In B. M. Melnyk & E. Fineout-Overholt (Eds.), *Evidence-based practice in nursing & healthcare: A guide to best practice* (3rd ed.) (pp. 376–388). Philadelphia, PA: Wolters Kluwer.

Fineout-Overholt, E., Levin, R., & Melnyk, B. M. (2004/2005). Strategies for advancing evidence-based practice in clinical settings. *Journal of the New York State Nurses Association, 35*(2), 28–32.

Gifford, W., Davies, B., Edwards, N., Griffin, P., & Lybanon, V. (2007). Managerial leadership for nurses' use of research evidence: An integrative review of the literature. *Worldviews on Evidence-Based Nursing, 4*(3), 126–145.

Levin, R. F., Fineout-Overholt, E., Melnyk, B. M., Barnes, M., & Vetter, M. J. (2011). Fostering evidence-based practice to improve nurse and cost outcomes in a community health setting: A pilot test of the advancing research and clinical practice through close collaboration model. *Nursing Administration Quarterly, 35*(1), 21–33.

Melnyk, B. M. (2012). Achieving a high-reliability organization through implementation of the ARCC model for system wide sustainability of evidence-based practice. *Nursing Administration Quarterly, 36*(2), 127–135.

Melnyk, B. M. (2014a). Building cultures and environments that facilitate clinician behavior change to evidence-based practice: What works? *Worldviews on Evidence-Based Nursing, 11*(2), 79–80.

Melnyk, B. M. (2014b). Speeding the translation of research into evidence-based practice and conducting projects that impact healthcare quality, patient outcomes and costs: The "so what" outcome factors. *Worldviews on Evidence-Based Nursing, 11*(1), 1–4.

Melnyk, B. M., & Fineout-Overholt, E. (2003). The Evidence-based Practice Beliefs Scale and the Evidence-based Practice Implementation Scale. Phoenix, Arizona: ARCC, LLC.

Melnyk, B. M., & Fineout-Overholt, E. (2015). *Evidence-based practice in nursing & healthcare: A guide to best practice* (3rd ed.). Philadelphia, PA: Wolters Kluwer.

Melnyk, B. M., Fineout-Overholt, E., Giggleman, M., & Cruz, R. (2010). Correlates among cognitive beliefs, EBP implementation, organizational culture, cohesion and job satisfaction in evidence-based practice mentors from a community hospital system. *Nursing Outlook, 58*(6), 301–308.

Melnyk, B. M., Fineout-Overholt, E., & Mays, M. Z. (2008). The evidence-based practice beliefs and implementation scales: Psychometric properties of two new instruments. *Worldviews on Evidence-Based Nursing, 5*(4), 208–216.

Melnyk, B. M., & Gallagher-Ford, L. (2014). Evidence-based practice as mission critical for healthcare quality and safety: A disconnect for many nurse executives. *Worldviews on Evidence-Based Nursing, 11*(3), 145–146.

Melnyk, B. M., Fineout-Overholt, E., Gallagher-Ford, L., & Kaplan, L. (2012). The state of evidence-based practice in US nurses: Critical implications for nurse leaders and educators. *Journal of Nursing Administration, 42*(9), 410–417.

Melnyk, B. M., Gallagher-Ford, L., Long, L. E., & Fineout-Overholt, E. (2014). The establishment of evidence-based practice competencies for practicing registered nurses and advanced practice nurses in real-world clinical settings: Proficiencies to improve healthcare quality, reliability, patient outcomes, and costs. *Worldviews on Evidence-Based Nursing, 11*(1), 5–15.

Melnyk, B. M., Gallagher-Ford, L., Koshy, B. K., Troseth, M., Wyngarden, K., & Szalacha, L. (2016). A study of chief nurse executives indicates low prioritization of evidence-based practice and shortcomings in hospital performance metrics across the United States. *Worldviews on Evidence-Based Nursing, 11*(1), 5–15.

Rogers, E. M. (2003). *Diffusion of innovations* (5th ed.). New York, NY: The Free Press.

Rycroft-Malone, J., Seers, K., Chandler, J., Hawkes, C. A., Crichton, N., Allen, C., . . . Strunin, L. (2013). The role of evidence, context, and facilitation in an implementation trial: Implications for the development of the PARIHS framework. *Implementation Science, 9*:8–28. doi:10.1186/1748-5908-8-28

Sredl, D., Melnyk, B. M., Hsueh, K.-H., Jenkins, R., Ding, C. D., & Durham, J. (2010). Health care in crisis. Can nurse executives' beliefs about and implementation of evidence-based practice be key solutions in health care reform? *Teaching and Learning in Nursing, 6*(2), 73–79.

Stetler, C. B., Ritchie, J. A., Rycroft-Malone, J., & Charns, M. P. (2014). Leadership for evidence-based practice: Strategic and functional behaviors for institutionalizing EBP. *Worldviews on Evidence-Based Nursing, 11*(4), 219–226.

Titler, M. G., Kleiber, C., Steelman, V., Rakel, B. A., Budreau, G., Everett, L. Q., . . . Goode, C. J. (2001). The Iowa model of evidence-based practice to promote quality care. *Critical Care Nursing Clinics of North America, 13*(4), 497–509.

Wallen, G. R., Mitchell, S. A., Melnyk, B. M., Fineout-Overholt, E., Miller-Davis, C., Yates, J., & Hastings, C. (2010). Implementing evidence-based practice: Effectiveness of a structured multifaceted mentorship programme. *Journal of Advanced Nursing, 66*(12), 2761–2771.

THE EVIDENCE-BASED PRACTICE COMPETENCIES RELATED TO DISSEMINATING EVIDENCE

Bernadette Mazurek Melnyk, PhD, RN, CPNP/PMHNP, FAANP, FNAP, FAAN

KEY CONTENT IN THIS CHAPTER

- The importance of disseminating evidence

- Various strategies to disseminate evidence

- Evidence-based practice competencies #12 and #24

- Strategies for meeting competencies for disseminating evidence

- Assessment of EBP competencies for disseminating evidence

> "Success is stumbling from failure to failure with no loss of enthusiasm."
>
> –Winston S. Churchill

SETTING THE STAGE

An interprofessional team of nurses, physicians, and physical therapists who practice together on a medical surgical unit were troubled by an increase in falls in their older adult patients over the past year and wondered whether there was a more effective evidence-based strategy that they could implement to decrease the fall rate (Step #0 in the EBP process). Therefore, they asked the following PICOT question (Step #1 in the EBP process):

In hospitalized older adults (P), how does an evidence-based fall protocol (I) compared to standard care (C) reduce fall rates (O) 12 months after implementation (T)?

After searching for the evidence to answer their PICOT question and critically appraising it (Steps #2 and #3 in the EBP process), they decided to implement an evidence-based protocol to reduce falls on their unit (Step #4 in the EBP process). Educational sessions for all staff on this medical-surgical unit were held to teach the new protocol. Twelve months following implementation of the new protocol, the team evaluated the outcome of their practice change and were very pleased to report to their nurse manager that the fall rate of their older adult patients had declined to nearly zero after implementing the protocol 12 months ago (Step #5 in the EBP process). However, they did not share these findings with anyone beyond their unit, and the fall rates of older adult patients remained high throughout the rest of the hospital.

THE IMPORTANCE OF DISSEMINATING EVIDENCE

The preceding scenario is all-too-common in healthcare systems across the United States. Clinicians often make evidence-based practice (EBP) decisions or changes that improve outcomes in their patients but fail to communicate their successes to others. As a result, Step #6 in the EBP process—disseminate the outcomes of the

EBP decision or change—does not occur, and others do not benefit from evidence-based changes that could result in a higher quality of care and improved patient outcomes.

Strategies for Disseminating Evidence

The primary goal of disseminating evidence is to increase the adoption of research findings into practice to ultimately improve patient outcomes (Majid et al., 2011). Mechanisms for disseminating evidence include unit-based short clinical presentations, grand rounds, or written summaries to colleagues at work; oral or poster presentations at local, regional, and national/international conferences; newsletter and journal publications; and the media. Even before an EBP change is made, thoughtful consideration should be given to whom and where the outcomes of the project will be disseminated so that others can learn about or benefit from the work.

Disseminating Evidence to Colleagues

You have a variety of opportunities with which to share evidence with colleagues at work, including the informal sharing of new evidence-based guidelines or recently published studies. The National Guideline Clearinghouse is one public resource for evidence-based clinical practice guidelines.

Although it is important to share the best and latest evidence-based guidelines and studies with colleagues, EBP changes made to improve healthcare quality and patient outcomes will require more than the passive dissemination of information because this strategy alone does not usually result in a change in others' behaviors (Melnyk, 2014). All EBP changes and quality improvement projects based on the best evidence require a solid plan for implementation and evaluation (see Chapter 6 for strategies on implementing an evidence-based practice change and Chapter 7 for outcomes evaluation).

NATIONAL GUIDELINE CLEARINGHOUSE

The National Guideline Clearinghouse is an initiative of the Agency for Healthcare Research and Quality (AHRQ) with a mission to provide healthcare professionals, health plans, integrated delivery systems, and others an accessible mechanism for obtaining objective, detailed information on clinical practice guidelines and furthering their dissemination, implementation, and use. The guidelines are easily searchable by topic. You can find more information at https://www.guideline.gov.

Onsite and online journal clubs are wonderful venues in which to share best evidence and increase the EBP knowledge and skills levels of clinicians in small groups. Advanced practice nurses (APNs) typically serve as the lead for a journal club until other nurses have the EBP skills to lead a group. Success of journal clubs depends upon a variety of factors, including expertise of the leader in selecting articles that provide pertinent sources of evidence, access to resources that facilitate activities of the journal club (e.g., searchable databases such as the Cochrane Database of Systematic Reviews, MEDLINE, and CINAHL), engagement by participants, demonstrated practice changes based on the work conducted in the journal club, and topics of clinical interest and relevance (Betz, Smith, Melnyk, & Olbrysh, 2015). For a full description on how to conduct onsite and online journal clubs, see Betz et al., 2015.

Evidence-based practice grand rounds are another mechanism for disseminating evidence to a group of colleagues. Many hospitals and healthcare systems offer these as an opportunity to share the outcomes of EBP implementation or quality improvement (QI) projects and research studies as well as evidence-based recommendations for changes in practice based on a thorough review of a body of evidence. Grand rounds usually involve formal oral presentations followed by a question and answer interchange with colleagues.

Evidence-based clinical rounds—which are smaller in scope and less formal than grand rounds—are often conducted on patient units. However, they can be a very effective medium for disseminating evidence to a small group of colleagues to ultimately guide clinical practice changes. These more informal rounds can be accomplished in 20 to 30 minutes and typically include the following:

- Background on the clinical problem

- The PICOT question

- The search process used to answer the PICOT question

- A succinct summary of the evidence with a critical appraisal of its quality

- Recommendations for practice change(s) based upon the evidence

- A plan to evaluate outcomes of the practice change(s)

Hospital/organizational and professional committee meetings provide another medium in which to share best evidence to change practice and are often part of a larger process necessary to make system-wide practice changes throughout a hospital or organization. In preparation for the meeting, determine who will be attending the meeting, including their roles, issues that are important to address for the committee, preference for type of presentation (e.g., a formal presentation with slides versus an informal presentation with a handout and discussion), and time allocation to make the presentation and answer questions. Committee meetings typically have tight time frames, so strive to not exceed the time allotment given.

Oral Presentations at Local, Regional, and National Conferences

Oral presentations at local, regional, and national conferences are an excellent strategy with which to disseminate EBP implementation and QI projects as well as findings from research studies. In preparation to make an oral presentation, you need to:

- Understand the audience who will be attending the presentation.

- Follow the conference guidelines for the presentation, including use of audiovisual materials and time allotment.

- Adhere to the time allotted for the presentation, especially if you are part of a panel of speakers so that your presentation does not shorten the next speaker's time frame.

If using PowerPoint slides as part of your presentation, make sure the slides are engaging and easy to read. An error that many novice presenters make is placing too much information on the slides, making it difficult for the audience to read them. Some tips for optimal presentations are:

- Use simple fonts, with the font size large enough to read. The Arial font, at 24 and 32 points, is very readable.

- Pick a background color and use it consistently throughout the presentation, with bolded headings. A dark background color (e.g., black or navy blue) with light lettering (e.g., white or yellow) works well. As another option, you can use dark lettering (e.g., black or navy blue) on a white background.

- Enhance the text with visuals (photos and graphs).

Many excellent examples of how to create outstanding PowerPoint presentations are freely available on the Internet, including the National Conference of State Legislatures at http://www.ncsl.org/legislators-staff/legislative-staff/legislative-staff-coordinating-committee/tips-for-making-effective-powerpoint-presentations.

As you develop each slide in your presentation, ask yourself, "What are the one or two most important points that I want to convey on this slide?" A good rule is to use one slide, but no more than two, for each minute of allocated time for the presentation. Therefore, for a 20-minute presentation, using 20 slides would be ideal.

For an EBP implementation or QI project presentation, the following content is suggested:

- Background of the problem

- The PICOT question

- Search strategy (e.g., the databases used) and the evidence that was found (e.g., the number and types of studies)

- Critical appraisal, evaluation, and synthesis of the evidence from the search

- The practice change that was made based on the evidence search

- Outcomes resulting from the evidence-based change or QI project

- Recommendations for future practice and research if applicable

 After your talk is completed, a great goal is to make a commitment to write the presentation in manuscript form and submit it for publication within 90 days. Because so much time and effort were invested into preparing the oral presentation, you have a wonderful foundation for a manuscript.

Poster Presentations

Poster presentations afford another excellent opportunity to share evidence at local, regional, and national conferences. Do not be disappointed if your abstract is accepted for a poster presentation instead of an oral presentation because posters are an outstanding venue with which to disseminate EBP and QI projects. Plus, the advantage of poster presentations is that they provide an opportunity to have one-to-one exchanges with conference participants in a more intimate fashion than what is possible in a formal oral presentation.

When preparing a poster, remember to follow directions that were provided to a "tee." Sketching out your ideas first in a mock-up poster either on paper with poster notes or on a computer template is helpful (Hamilton, 2008). Typical EBP implementation and QI project poster presentations include:

- Title and authors

- Background of the problem or clinical issue

- The PICOT question

 Be excited, not discouraged, when you have an abstract accepted for a poster presentation!

- The search process (e.g., the databases used and number of studies found)

- Critical appraisal, evaluation, and synthesis of the evidence

- The practice change that was made based upon the evidence

- Evaluation of outcomes that resulted from the EBP change

- Implications for further clinical practice

In creating the poster, remember to:

- Make it visually appealing with photographs and graphs while limiting the amount of wording to text blocks of 50 or fewer words, with short sentences of 7 words or fewer (Betz et al., 2015).

- Use 100-point font for your title; headings should be large and bold with 36- to 48-point font.

- Avoid using underlining, and limit references.

- Organize the text for reading: left to right and top to bottom.

Have small prints of the poster with your contact information so that individuals can reach you if they have further questions about your work.

Most conferences require poster presenters to stand beside their posters for the entire time of the poster session.

You can find many helpful websites to create outstanding posters, including https://www.ncsu.edu/project/posters/ and http://www.free-power-point-templates.com/articles/create-poster-powerpoint-2010. After the poster presentation is completed, make it a goal to write and submit a manuscript that captures the essence of the material presented for journal publication within 90 days so that others can learn and benefit from your EBP project.

Publications

Publication all starts with the vision of what you want to publish: for example, an EBP implementation or QI project, an evidence review, or an editorial. Start a creative ideas publishing file that you can refer to when you have some time to begin a manuscript so that you do not lose great potential manuscripts. Think about your target audience (e.g., clinicians, nurse managers/executives, or the public), specifically where you would like your manuscript published (e.g., a clinical nursing journal, a journal for nurse managers or executives, a public newspaper), and how fast you would like to see it in print (production time from acceptance of the manuscript to publication is variable). Although not always required, sometimes it is helpful to contact the editor of a journal to inquire about potential interest in your proposed paper. Inform the editor of your idea for the manuscript and why you believe the journal would be interested in it. Also include an abstract of what you are proposing to write. Most editors will respond affirmatively to your inquiry, which is why it is not necessary to take this step in the manuscript submission process.

If you are a novice writer, find a mentor who has experience in publishing: someone with a good publication record and a compatible personality and writing style. Seek someone who can provide you with constructive—not destructive—feedback.

When planning the manuscript, use other articles that have been published as a template. Sketch out a plan and outline for the manuscript and think about the following:

- What is my main message?

- What did I do?

- How did I do it?

- What did I find?

- What are the implications?

If you are writing a paper with colleagues, author credit should be based on their contributions, which can include helping to conceive the article, conducting the evaluation of outcomes/data analysis, interpreting the data, drafting sections of the article or helping with revisions, and reviewing the final draft with suggestions for improvement. Discuss with your writing colleagues openly and honestly upfront to agree upon the order of authorship as well as what each author will contribute to the paper prior to commencing the written work to avoid later problems.

> *Remember: You never get a second chance to make a great first impression, so make the first submission of the manuscript as flawless as possible.* —Bernadette Melnyk

Do the very best job that you can in writing the manuscript the first time—after all, you never get a second chance to make a great first impression with the reviewers. Journals publish author guidelines on their website, and you must absolutely follow those directions to a "tee." If the word limit of manuscripts is 4,000 words, do not exceed that limit. Various journals have different requirements, so follow them carefully. More clinically focused journals, such as the *American Journal of Nursing* and *Worldviews on Evidence-Based Nursing*, publish EBP implementation and QI projects. *Worldviews* has a regular column for these types of manuscripts entitled *Implementing and Sustaining EBP in Real World Practice Settings*, which uses the seven steps of EBP as the template for papers.

Turn to Chapter 1 for the seven steps of EBP.

For evidence-review manuscripts, the following content is recommended:

- Introduction, including significance of the problem

- The PICOT question

- Search for the evidence, with search strategy and databases searched

- Evidence found with critical appraisal of the evidence (it is helpful to table the studies)

- Implications for clinical practice and further research

Additional tips for writing manuscripts include:

- Have an editor or someone with expertise in publishing review your paper for content, grammar, style, and clarity.

- Prepositions are not words to end sentences *with*.

- Avoid using abbreviations.

- Avoid redundancy.

- Spell-check the document before submission and read it thoroughly to detect errors.

Most journals are *peer-reviewed*, meaning that submissions are usually reviewed and critiqued by at least two or three reviewers. To help prevent bias, authors' names are removed from the papers before they are sent to the reviewers, and authors do not know who reviewed their manuscripts. Typical review criteria usually include:

- Ideas and information in the manuscript are innovative and important.

- The content expands the readers' knowledge and skills.

- The content is relevant to the readers.

- The content is applicable to practice.

- The paper is well written and organized.

- Content is clear and flows logically.

- Methods are appropriate.

- Findings are clearly presented.

- Conclusions are sound.

- References are current (within the past 3 to 5 years unless important older landmark studies need cited).

Along with their critique of the manuscript for strengths and limitations, reviewers should provide suggestions on how the manuscript can be improved. Authors usually receive feedback on their submitted paper within 2 to 3 months of their submissions. There are three possible scenarios that result from the review: the paper is accepted (which rarely happens on the first try); you are asked to revise and resubmit; or the paper is rejected.

Typical reasons for rejection include that the content is not new, a similar paper was recently published, the guidelines were not followed, or the writing style is not clear (a fatal flaw). If a paper was rejected because a particular journal has a similar paper already, query another journal that might be interested in publishing your work, but do not give up. Very few papers are accepted without revisions. Additionally, many well-written papers are rejected because the content and focus would be better suited to another journal. Remember that *the paper is not you*. Even if you are shocked, disappointed, and/or stressed if your paper is rejected, read the comments and critiques and then put them aside for a few days while your emotions are running high until you can read with more objectivity.

If you are asked to revise the paper, address each reviewer's comments and suggestions. Although you do not have to agree with all of them, you should be sensitive to most of them and provide strong rationale if you decide not to follow a suggestion by the reviewers. Most journals ask for you to describe how you responded to each of the reviewers' comments in the cover letter that accompanies the revised paper. In addition, journals often ask to see the changes you made in the paper through word-processor tracked changes or highlighted font.

If you decide not to resubmit the paper to the same journal, sending a letter to the editor explaining your decision is professional courtesy.

After revising your paper, but before resubmitting, have experienced authors read the revised manuscript. Providing them with a copy of the reviewers' critique is helpful so they can assess whether you have addressed all of the concerns and suggestions from the review.

Successful publishing requires you to stay focused on your dream (disseminating important work) and block uninterrupted time to write regularly. It also requires that you persist in writing and rewriting the work that you believe is important for others to learn about and benefit from.

The Media and Lay Publications

Consider sharing evidence with the media and through lay publications so that the public is aware of best evidence. Clinicians tend to focus heavily on disseminating their work through professional conferences and in journals, but they often do not think about the media and lay publications as important outlets.

The first step in obtaining media attention is to craft an "elevator message"— something newsworthy and easy to understand. For example, effective elevator messages that would probably capture media attention would be, "Behaviors are the #1 killer of Americans" or "Sitting is the new smoking." Using something like, "Cardiovascular disease is the leading cause of mortality in the U.S." is certainly true but does not have the media appeal of the former examples.

Think about the audience that you would like to reach before you craft your message. Use your public relations or media office if one exists to assist you in reaching out to media because they will likely have already established relationships with reporters. Your media office can also help you draft a press release to capture the evidence that you believe is important to share with the public. Reporters often are on overload with a heaping plate of incoming stories of what people believe to be newsworthy, so established relationships with known entities can be helpful in succeeding with media attention.

Lay journals, such as *Prevention* or *Parents* magazine, are other outlets to share best evidence with the public. A personal communication with the editors of these types of journals that outlines the type of evidence-based story that you would like to share is often the best strategy to determine whether they have any interest in publishing it. Stories in these types of publications need to be written in lay language that is relatable and understandable for the general public.

Briefs for Policy Change

Another venue is to create health policy issue briefs with concisely presented evidence on issues that you consider important for health policy change as well as changes to policies within your healthcare organization. Policy briefs can be effective tools to provide best evidence on a topic that can influence important health policy or organizational policy issues. Professional organizations, such as the American Academy of Nursing, frequently publishes policy briefs in its journal *Nursing Outlook*. *Health Affairs* is another journal that publishes policy briefs. Hospitals and healthcare systems also typically have policy and procedure manuals in which briefs are published. Formatting the brief as follows is suggested:

- The title that conveys the brief's purpose

- Clear statement of the policy issue (e.g., lack of mental health services for children and teens)

- Context and background of the issue/problem (consider using concise bullets denoting the information and relevant data)

- Options: pros and cons of each recommendation offered

- Resources used to prepare the policy brief

 # COMPETENCY #12

Disseminates best practices supported by evidence
to improve quality of care and patient outcomes.

Strategies for Implementing Competency #12

- Stay current with best practices to improve care and outcomes for patients through a variety of venues (e.g., searching for best evidence; reading journal articles, accessing the National Guideline Clearinghouse and other evidence-based guideline databases; attending seminars, grand rounds, and continuing education offerings; participating in EBP fellowship programs and journal clubs).

- Share best practices with colleagues through verbal and/or written communications.

Assessment of Competency #12

Is the RN or APN able to:

- Stay current with best practices as evidenced by searching for best evidence and seeking opportunities to update knowledge of best practices by such venues as attending continuing education conferences and grand rounds/EBP presentations, participating in journal clubs, and engaging in EBP initiatives.

- Share best practices with colleagues through formal or informal written or verbal communications.

COMPETENCY #24

Communicates best evidence to individuals, groups, colleagues, and policy makers.

Strategies for Implementing Competency #24

- Routinely update staff and administration on best practices to improve healthcare quality and patient outcomes.

- Inform patients of best evidence when treatment or care decisions are being made.

- Develop a plan for communicating evidence to specific target audiences at the outset of EBP implementation or quality improvement projects (i.e., to whom will the evidence be communicated and how).

- Communicate best evidence to policy makers within and external to the healthcare system through oral and written communications when indicated.

- Work with the public relations office if one exists or directly with the media to communicate best evidence.

- Develop abstracts from EBP or QI projects that have been implemented.

- Submit abstracts to professional conferences.

- Make EBP oral and/or poster presentations at local, regional, and national events.

- Participate in writing manuscripts for professional journals that are published.

Assessment of Competency #24

Is the APN able to:

- Share best practices routinely with staff and administration.

- Inform patients of the best evidence when making treatment or care decisions.

- Develop a plan for communicating evidence to specific target audiences at the outset of EBP implementation or QI projects.

- Communicate best evidence to policy makers within and external to the healthcare system through oral and written communications when indicated.

- Work with the public relations office if one exists or directly with the media to communicate best evidence.

- Submit abstracts for presentation at professional conferences.

- Make quality EBP oral and/or poster presentations at local, regional, and national events.

- Participate in writing manuscripts that are published in professional journals.

A REAL-WORLD EXAMPLE

MEETING COMPETENCIES #12 AND #24

Logan is a seasoned school nurse who works at one of six high schools in an urban school district in the Midwest. He is troubled by the fact that he is seeing a rise in both obesity and depression in the teens at his school and wonders whether there are evidence-based intervention programs that could be implemented to address these public health issues (Step #0 in the EBP process). Logan remembers reading an article last month that described the benefits of using cognitive-behavioral therapy–based (CBT) interventions for both depression and obesity in adolescents, so he asks the following PICOT question (Step #1 in the EBP process):

In high school teens (P), how do CBT–based interventions (I) compared to interventions that are not based on CBT (C) affect obesity and depression (O) 6 and 12 months after the intervention (T)?

His search for evidence yielded only two recently published papers. The first described the outcomes from a randomized controlled trial by Melnyk and colleagues (2013) that evaluated a 15-session cognitive-behavioral skills-building intervention entitled the COPE (Creating Opportunities for Personal Empowerment) Healthy Lifestyles TEEN (Thinking, Emotions, Exercise, and Nutrition) Program (Step #2 in the EBP process) on the healthy lifestyle behaviors, body mass index (BMI), and mental health outcomes of high school teens. Findings from this study indicated that teens who received the intervention program versus those who received an attention-control program had higher levels of physical activity, less incidence of being overweight/obesity, higher social skills, less alcohol use, and higher grade performance 6 months after the intervention. At 12 months following the intervention program, COPE teens who were severely depressed at baseline had symptoms that decreased into the normal range versus teens

continues

continued

who received the attention-control program. The second study yielded that additionally, teens in the intervention program group had less incidence of being overweight/obesity than the attention-control group teens (Melnyk et al., 2015). Logan critically appraised the study and found it to be valid, reliable, and applicable to practice (Step #3 in the EBP process).

At the next district-wide school nurses meeting, Logan asked Kaylin, his master's prepared director of school nursing, whether he could make a brief presentation to the other school nurses on the evidence that he found, with the suggestion that they embark on a small-scale EBP change project to deliver the intervention to a classroom in three of their high schools. Two other nurses got excited about the evidence that Logan presented and the opportunity to improve these outcomes in their high school teens. Kaylin also was excited about the project and was eager to mentor Logan and the other two nurses in conducting an EBP implementation project. She scheduled a separate follow-up meeting for the three school nurses to make a plan to implement and evaluate the program at their three high schools (Step #4 in the EBP process).

At the start of the next school year, Logan and his two colleagues provided the COPE program to 30 students in a health class at each of their high schools. At the end of the school year, they were delighted to find similar outcomes as were reported in the original intervention program trial (Step #5 in the EBP process). Kaylin helped the three nurses to submit an abstract for an oral presentation at the upcoming National Association of School Nurses conference. To their delight, the abstract was accepted for an oral presentation. Following the conference, Kaylin mentored the three nurses in writing a manuscript that described their project. The paper was accepted in the *Implementing and Sustaining EBP in Real World Practice Settings* column in *Worldviews on Evidence-Based Nursing* (Step #6 in the EBP process).

SUMMARY

After conducting an EBP or QI project, it is important to disseminate the outcomes through various venues such as presentations at conferences and publications in journals or lay media venues. Disseminating evidence assists others in learning various strategies that can improve outcomes in their own healthcare settings.

REFERENCES

Betz, C. L., Smith, K. N., Melnyk, B. M., & Olbrysh, T. (2015). Disseminating evidence through publications, presentations, health policy briefs, and the media. In B. M. Melnyk & E. Fineout-Overholt (Eds.), *Evidence-based practice in nursing & healthcare: A guide to best practice* (pp. 391–431). Philadelphia, PA: Wolters Kluwer.

Hamilton, C. W. (2008). At a glance: A stepwise approach to successful poster presentations. *Chest, 134,* 457–459.

Majid, S., Foo, S., Luyt, B., Zhang, X., Theng, Y., Chang, Y., & Mokhtar, I. (2011). Adopting evidence-based practice in clinical decision making: Nurses' perceptions, knowledge, and barriers. *Journal of the Medical Library Association, 99*(3), 229–236.

Melnyk, B. M. (2014). Building cultures and environments that facilitate clinician behavior change to evidence-based practice: What works? *Worldviews on Evidence-Based Nursing, 11*(2), 79–80.

Melnyk, B. M., Jacobson, D., Kelly, S., Belyea, M., Shaibi, G., Small, L., … Marsiglia, F. F. (2013). Promoting healthy lifestyles in high school adolescents: A randomized controlled trial. *American Journal of Preventive Medicine, 45*(4), 407–415.

Melnyk, B. M., Jacobson, D., Kelly, S. A., Belyea, M. J., Shaibi, G. Q., Small, L., … Marsiglia, F. F. (2015). Twelve-month effects of the COPE Healthy Lifestyles TEEN program on overweight and depressive symptoms in high school adolescents. *Journal of School Health, 85*(12), 861–870.

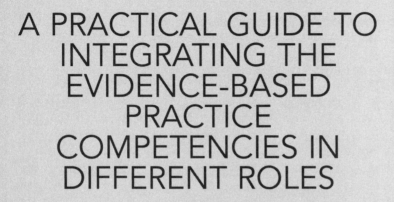

A PRACTICAL GUIDE TO INTEGRATING THE EVIDENCE-BASED PRACTICE COMPETENCIES IN DIFFERENT ROLES

Chapters 10–13 outline how to integrate the evidence-based practice competencies in healthcare settings, the advanced practice nurse role, policy and procedure committees, and clinical and academic settings.

Chapter 10. 185

Chapter 11. 205

Chapter 12. 225

Chapter 13. 245

INTEGRATING THE EVIDENCE-BASED PRACTICE COMPETENCIES IN HEALTHCARE SETTINGS

Lynn Gallagher-Ford, PhD, RN, DPFNAP, NE-BC

KEY CONTENT IN THIS CHAPTER

- Strategies for integrating evidence-based practice (EBP) competencies in healthcare settings

- Return on investment (ROI) of integrating EBP competencies in healthcare settings

- Using EBP competencies to develop educational programs

- Using EBP competencies for interprofessional learning and collaboration

- Benefits of integrating the EBP competencies in clinical settings

> It's hard to beat a person who never gives up.
>
> –*Babe Ruth*

Competence is often described as a concept that incorporates knowledge, skills and attitudes, and the capability to do something well (Ilic, 2009; Melnyk, Gallagher-Ford, Long, & Fineout-Overholt, 2014). Competencies are holistic entities that are carried out within clinical contexts and are composed of multiple attributes including knowledge, psychomotor skills, and affective skills. Dunn and colleagues (2000, p. 341) contended that competency is not a "skill or task to be done, but characteristics required in order to act effectively in the nursing setting." Although a particular competency "cannot exist without scientific knowledge, clinical skills, and humanistic values" (Dunn et al., 2000, p. 341), the actual competency transcends each of the individual components. A variety of health professions have used competencies as a mechanism to determine whether clinicians are providing high-quality safe care (Gallagher-Ford, Buck, & Melnyk, 2014).

Measurement of nurses' competencies related to various patient care activities is a standard ongoing activity in a multitude of healthcare organizations across the globe, and now, with the arrival of these user-friendly, research-based EBP competencies, measurement of knowledge, skills, and attitudes in evidence-based practice can be achieved. The EBP competencies serve as the tool needed to help individuals and organizations to integrate evidence-based thinking and decision-making into daily practice. Because the competencies clearly describe in measurable terms what every clinician needs to know and needs to do to be evidence-based in their practice, it becomes realistic to create expectations and measure performance. Now that these are available, leaders are equipped with the tool needed to take action and move their organizations toward evidence-based, high-quality, and safe care.

STRATEGIES FOR INTEGRATING THE EBP COMPETENCIES IN HEALTHCARE SETTINGS

To achieve high-quality and safe care, EBP competence expectations cannot be integrated haphazardly; they must be a performance expectation of every nurse in the organization—they cannot be an option. Evidence-based practice competence must be expected regardless of the nurses' level of education, years of experience, tenure in a particular organization, or novice versus expert status.

For the integration of the EBP competencies to have the biggest impact, they must be embedded in multiple ways and through a variety of mechanisms that affect every practicing nurse in the organization. Examples of mechanisms include mission statements, job descriptions, development of EBP mentors, ladder programs, shared governance councils, policy and procedure committees, and explicit leadership role requirements.

Mission Statements

A powerful way to establish the nursing enterprise's commitment to EBP is to state it clearly in the departmental mission—the document that expresses the core intentions and values of nurses throughout the organization. The following sidebar shows a mission statement, with language that addresses EBP in bold.

PROFESSIONAL NURSING PRACTICE MISSION

The professional practice of nursing combines scientific precision with empathy in caring for and nurturing of patients. Nurses thrive in an environment that promotes **clinical inquiry, and inclusion of best evidence, clinical expertise, and patient voice** to underpin our care. Excellence in nursing practice is based on lifelong learning, effective communication, and autonomy in practice. Nurses provide the highest level of quality-driven, patient-centered care **utilizing current evidence-based knowledge and skills.** Nurses fulfill this responsibility by assuring their education is ongoing, working collaboratively with physicians and other members of the healthcare team, and actively participating in autonomous decision-making related to their practice.

Job Descriptions

Integration of the EBP competencies in tangible, operational processes such as onboarding/orientation and job descriptions/performance appraisals reflects the organization's explicit commitment to EBP from the moment of hire and every day thereafter. A job description for an RN that incorporates EBP might look like the following; the EBP-centric language is in bold:

- Establish a compassionate environment by providing emotional, psychological, and spiritual support to patients, friends, and families.

- **Participate in EBP by questioning practices to improve care, describing clinical problems using evidence, participating in the steps of the EBP process, and promoting a culture of EBP.**

- **Participate in research activities when appropriate.**

- Promote patient independence by establishing patient care goals; teaching patient and family to understand condition, medications, and self-care skills; and answering questions.

- Assure quality of care by adhering to nursing ethics and standards; measuring health outcomes against patient care goals and standards; **making evidence-based recommendations;** and following hospital and nursing division's philosophies and standards of care set by state board of nursing, state nurse practice act, and other governing agency regulations.

- Resolve patient problems and needs by using multidisciplinary team strategies.

- Promote a safe and positive working environment.

- Maintain continuity of care by documenting and communicating actions, irregularities, and continuing needs.

- Maintain patient confidence and protect operations by keeping information confidential.

- Maintain professional competence (knowledge, skills, and attitudes) by attending ongoing educational programs, reviewing professional publications, establishing personal networks, and participating in professional organization(s).

- Communicate effectively with healthcare team members by active participation in clinical discussions, communicating information, responding to requests, building rapport, and participating in team problem-solving.

EBP Mentors

Creating specific EBP mentor positions is a powerful strategy that organizations have implemented to effectively build an EBP program and deliver a strong message about the organization's commitment to establishing EBP as part of day-to-day operations. A job description that reflects the EBP competencies created specifically for the EBP mentor provides a clear articulation of their role, responsibilities, and deliverables. It creates a framework for an ongoing EBP program and designates the mentor's accountability to projects implemented and outcomes achieved. An EBP mentor job description would include:

- Manage time effectively, able to function independently and autonomously.

- Stimulate, facilitate, and educate nursing staff and healthcare providers toward an EBP culture.

- Actively participate in and coach others' ongoing clinical inquiry.

- Foster critical thinking about clinical issues to encourage nurses' use of research findings in making clinical decisions.

- Develop and implement evidence-based projects.

- Provide comprehensive EBP support to staff and colleagues: formulating PICOT questions, conducting searches, evaluating and synthesizing a body of evidence, and making recommendations for practice changes.

- Anticipate and navigate barriers to evidence-based care through active engagement with organizational leadership.

- Collaborate with other healthcare providers in the integration of evidence in clinical decision-making.

- Conduct EBP rounds to bring the latest research findings from studies to nurses for implementation to improve patient outcomes.

- Generate internal evidence through quality improvement (QI) and outcomes-management programs.

- Participate in development of EBP guidelines, policies and procedures, and standards or practice models with integration of EBP.

- Provide leadership in attaining excellent clinical outcomes by acting as communication link and consultant to providers and other caregivers across departments, campuses, or systems.

- Lead transdisciplinary teams in applying synthesized evidence to initiate clinical decisions and practice changes to improve the health of individuals, groups, and populations.

- Coach others in evidence-based clinical decision-making, patient/family education, and problem-solving.

- Facilitate communication and promote collaborative behavior among team members. Mentor staff in effective communication techniques, conflict and crisis resolution, and team behaviors.

- Support and participate in research activities when there is not sufficient evidence to address clinical issues.

- Coordinate and participate in unit, multidepartment, or campus educational process in conjunction with educator, manager, and other experts.

- Assist in creation of strategic learning plans related to EBP for department and coordinate education delivery in conjunction with educator and manager.

- Participate in multidepartment, campus, and/or system task forces or committees.

- Teach EBP course twice per year or as needed.

- Serve as a consultant to other departments related to EBP.

- Actively participate in outside professional organization to advance patient care and for the nursing profession.

- Provide formal EBP–related presentations and/or posters at local or national venues.

- Assist nursing staff to disseminate evidence through regional and national presentations and peer-reviewed journals.

- Understand and guide others in Institutional Review Board (IRB) process.

Ladder Programs

In addition to the mechanisms that impact and reflect the performance of every nurse, EBP competencies can also be integrated in mechanisms that incentivize and acknowledge higher level attainment. By building the EBP competencies into systems such as clinical ladder programs or nursing leadership/advancement programs, nurses work toward becoming more proficient in their EBP knowledge and skills while they advance their careers. The following sidebar shows an example of a clinical ladder program that incorporates EBP; the EBP language is in bold.

CLINICAL LADDER PROGRAM FOR REGISTERED NURSES

Purpose:

To recognize and reward staff nurses for clinical expertise in delivering direct care to patients.

Offers:

An opportunity for career development/advancement while maintaining a clinical focus at point of care.

----

continues

continued

The Clinical Ladder program at XYZ Health System recognizes and rewards staff nurses for excellence in delivering direct care to patients. The participating RN is recognized with a promotion from Staff Nurse II to Staff Nurse III or IV and an increase in base salary. The Clinical Ladder program is a voluntary program in which the nurse demonstrates expertise in the areas of clinical management, educational activities, **evidence-based practice,** quality improvement, and research.

Examples of activities to demonstrate these areas include, but are not limited to:

- Serve on unit and hospital committees
- Demonstrate excellent patient care in complex situations
- Provide education to other healthcare providers
- Precept other staff members
- Participate in quality improvement initiatives
- **Participate in evidence-based practice projects**
- Participate in nursing research studies
- Achieve specialty certification

Shared Governance Councils

Other mechanisms that can be leveraged to promote integration of evidence-based thinking and decision-making might include requiring higher-level EBP competence expectations for clinicians interested in participating in shared governance councils. Not only is this another way to build EBP competence in the nursing enterprise, but it also enhances the probability that decisions and recommendations from all councils will be based in evidence, as opposed to tradition. Figure 10.1 shows a shared governance council charter with EBP; the EBP language is in bold.

XYZ Council Charter	Year One	Year Two	Comments
XYZ Council Name			
Demonstrate Attendance (80%)			
Demonstrate Participation in council projects			
Documentation of relevant ongoing education (XXX hours)			
Lead Role on Council Project:_____			
Evidence Integrated into Project			
Outcomes of Project reported/met ROI of project reported/met			
Dissemination of project completed			

Figure 10.1 Shared governance council charter.

Policy and Procedure Committees

Another innovative way to integrate the EBP competencies that provides an opportunity to expand their impact across multiple disciplines is requiring them as an expectation for members of policy and procedure committees. (See Chapter 12 for a discussion of this process.) Many organizations claim that their policies and procedures are evidence-based; however, upon close inspection, this claim is rarely legitimate. Often times, a policy/procedure has one or two references attached, which are considered "evidence," and there is no process (let alone a rigorous process) in place to gather, appraise, synthesize, or integrate the body of evidence to properly determine the best practice to be followed. This flawed approach, and the resulting flawed policies and procedures that are produced, can be remedied by integrating the EBP competencies as a requirement of all committee members.

Leadership Role Requirements

Another way to integrate the EBP competencies that have a deep impact is requiring the APN EBP competencies as expectations for nurses in leadership roles in the organization. Because it is so critical for leaders to create a supportive EBP environment, building nursing leaders' EBP knowledge and skills as well as their attitudes toward EBP can be a particularly powerful initiative to implement. Leadership roles come in many varieties, ranging from traditional roles with titles such as nurse executive, chief nursing officer, nursing director, nurse manager, assistant nurse manager, and charge nurse, to any number of more creative titles.

Regardless of title, the point is that if a nurse is functioning in a role that includes influencing the work environment where other nurses provide care, that nurse is in a leadership role. By creating the expectation that nurse leaders must have advanced EBP knowledge, skills, and attitudes, the message throughout the nursing enterprise is that EBP is taken seriously and is a top priority. Integrating the EBP competencies into leadership job descriptions and performance appraisal mechanisms clearly reflects an organization's commitment to evidence-based decision-making and practice from the c-suite (corporate suite) to the bedside—a powerful underpinning to building a culture of EBP. A leadership job description that incorporates EBP looks like this:

- **Job knowledge:** Demonstrates and uses skills and knowledge to effectively direct services in areas of responsibility.

  - Educates and mentors staff and leadership teams in EBP, research, and quality methodologies.

  - Role-models EBP in daily practice.

  - Assures integration of EBP, research, and quality processes across disciplines and the organization.

- **People management:** Recruits and hires employees to provide quality service in a manner consistent with XYZ Healthcare values.

    - Assembles effective EBP, research, and quality teams. Monitors effectiveness of teams and provides data-supported outcomes of teams' work.

    - Demonstrates ability to educate, train, and provide a healthy work environment that supports best (evidence-based) practices, best patient outcomes, and employee satisfaction.

- **Financial management:** Develops and controls department budget within xxx% of budget standards.

- Assures that all EBP, research, and quality projects include a business plan and estimated ROI prior to launch.

CALCULATING THE ROI OF EBP

When integrating EBP with any of these strategies, no new positions are being created. The workforce is not being expanded: It is being enriched.

Organizational investments that build knowledge and capacity in employees in meaningful ways serve not only the individual, but they enhance the organization as well.

Spending the time and effort to provide individuals with EBP education and support is an investment that has a tremendous potential return (ROI). As skilled EBP mentors are integrated into organizational operations, decision-making and care are more informed by current/best evidence, resulting in improved quality and safety outcomes, and ultimately, improved financial outcomes as well.

As many organizations have begun to integrate an evidence-based approach to decision-making and care across the healthcare enterprise, it is becoming ever clearer that this is the gold standard that drives quality and safety. As this paradigm begins to normalize in the healthcare industry, it will be risky business for an organization to ignore its obligation to build, support, and sustain an evidence-based enterprise. Not investing in creating an EBP enterprise will impact an even more important "ROI" in healthcare: *the risk of ignoring* what is known to be best for patients' families and the communities served.

Nurse Retention

Relevant, meaningful education can positively impact nursing satisfaction, recruitment, retention, and patient care and outcomes. In a study commissioned by the American Nurses Association in 2000, a direct correlation between staff retention and provision of quality educational initiatives was identified. Studies have demonstrated that professional development and education significantly affect commitment to the organization and the decision to remain at a particular hospital. For example, in 2004, Kramer and Schmalenberg found that staff satisfaction was strongly related to being able to provide good quality care, which was dependent on working with clinically competent and knowledgeable co-workers and the degree of organizational support provided for education and training. These authors also found that access to and support for educational opportunities was among the top eight job satisfiers for nurses.

When nurses participate in continuing professional development (CPD), a myriad of important attributes are built and enhanced. Studies in nursing have demonstrated that CPD increases their knowledge, supports professional competency, increases self-confidence, facilitates career development, improves the quality of care, and develops clinical decision-making skills (Covell, 2009; Hughes, 2005; Meyer, Paunonen, Gellatly, Goffin, & Jackson, 1989; Nolan, Owen, Curran, & Venables, 2000; and Wilcock, Janes, & Cambers, 2009).

Opportunities for professional development have been identified as an important strategy to retain nurses, especially those who are committed to the organization. *Affective commitment* refers to an individual's attachment to, identification with, and involvement in an organization. It reflects an individual's commitment to the goals and values of the organization and their intrinsic willingness to exert great effort on the organization's behalf. According to the literature, "commitment is a dynamic process of interaction between the person and his or her environment.

As employees become more involved in their organization, the nature of their commitment changes" (Liou, 2008, p. 119). When organizational commitment has been studied specifically in nursing, critical factors have included learning opportunities, job satisfaction, patient care, cultural factors, and relationship with co-workers. Affective commitment among employees improves the operational aspects of the organization. Its relationship to overall job satisfaction is significant in several studies (Gellaty, Cowden, & Cummings, 2014; Herscovitch & Meyer, 2002; Meyer et al., 1989). In addition, behaviors of good citizenship become more widespread, turnover rates fall, and employees have more opportunities to develop leadership skills.

Reducing Errors and Sentinel Events

A growing body of literature reflects that ongoing nursing education is a major influencing factor in reducing critical, nurse-sensitive quality indicators including medication errors, patient falls, pressure ulcers, and nosocomial infections (Aitken & Patrician, 2000; Shamian, 1997).

Continuing professional education and development can contribute to prevention of harm. The Joint Commission on Accreditation of Healthcare Organizations (2002) reported that 24% of *sentinel events* (events leading to mortality or morbidity) in the United States were related to inadequacy of professional and educational preparation and continuation of nursing staff for their roles. This is a completely avoidable situation. Organizations have the opportunity to build and deliver meaningful professional education and development programs for their clinicians.

Current evidence reflects that patients have better outcomes if they are cared for by more knowledgeable nurses, "a philosophy that views education (professional development) as an investment, fosters a hospital environment conducive to learning, facilitates the growth and development of its employees, and positively impacts patient outcomes" (Levett-Jones, 2005, p. 230).

EBP is extremely relevant and important content to offer through professional education/development for a variety of reasons—most importantly because EBP is correlated with improved patient outcomes—yet most clinicians currently in practice simply do not know what EBP is, let alone how to integrate evidence into their day-to-day practice. This is primarily related to the fact that the majority of clinicians currently in practice did not learn about EBP when they were in school. EBP content has only recently been integrated into many health sciences programs of study, and EBP is still not included or integrated into courses or across college curricula in many instances. People cannot be expected to do what they do not know, yet that is exactly what is happening in healthcare settings. Although the message from professional and regulatory agencies as well as organizational leadership is to: "integrate EBP," "do EBP," "demonstrate EBP," "provide exemplars of EBP," and so on, EBP is a low priority, and investment in building and supporting EBP programs is remarkably weak. These realities of the current "state of EBP" in healthcare organizations were demonstrated in a national survey of chief nursing officers/executives (CNOs/CNEs) in 2013, where 74% of CNOs and CNEs reported they spent between 0% and 10% of their budgets on EBP; EBP ranked as a low priority (only 3% of the CNOs/CNEs ranked EBP as a high priority); and CNOs/CNEs acknowledged they had inadequate numbers of EBP mentors in their organization to work on EBP with direct care staff and create EBP cultures/environments (Melnyk, Gallagher-Ford, & Troseth, 2016).

DEVELOPING EDUCATIONAL PROGRAMS AROUND THE EBP COMPETENCIES

EBP competencies can be used as a tool for conducting assessments of RN and APN knowledge and skills in EBP to identify gaps where targeted continuing education and skills-building workshops are needed. By surveying the staff on their self-assessed level of competence on each of the specific EBP competencies, educators can use the results to plan and implement targeted education strategies to build the knowledge and skills where gaps exist.

Rather than teaching everyone the same EBP knowledge and skills, the assessment survey (such as the one shown in Figure 10.2) can provide individualized or group information about what should be included in EBP education programs based on what nurses say they need. Here are some examples:

- In an organization with dedicated health sciences librarians, clinicians would likely assess their searching abilities higher than those of individuals working in organizations with no librarian(s). In the case where librarians are available, the targeted EBP education program would be designed to help clinicians learn how to access the librarians and how to prepare for working with the librarian, rather than how to conduct searches independently.

- In organizations with a strong partnership with an academic organization that provides access to PhD nurse scientists, clinicians would likely assess their ability to participate in the EBP and research processes as higher than those of individuals working in organizations with no access to nurse scientists. In the case where PhD nurse scientists are available, the targeted EBP education program would be tailored to emphasize how to access and work collaboratively with the nurse scientist(s) when a research study is indicated in the EBP process rather than how to initiate a process to conduct a research study (identifying a PhD nurse scientist to build a partnership with, developing a mechanism to support the partnership, etc.).

Regardless of the complexity of the organization and/or the robustness of the EBP program in place, the EBP competencies self-assessment survey can serve as a tool to better understand the current state of EBP in the organization, plan content for education programs to be offered, and develop short- and long-term strategies to support EBP activities throughout the organization.

Evidence-Based Practice Competencies for Practicing Registered Professional Nurses

Please identify your level of competence for each of the EBP competencies using the following 4-point Likert rating scale:

(1=Not Competent | 2=Need Improvement |3=Competent | 4=Highly Competent)

Competency	Not Competent 1	Need Improvement 2	Competent 3	Highly Competent 4
Competency 1: Questions clinical practices for the purpose of improving the quality of care.	O	O	O	O
Competency 2: Describes clinical problems using internal evidence* (*internal evidence = evidence generated internally within a clinical setting, such as patient assessment, outcomes management, and quality improvement data).	O	O	O	O
Competency 3: Participates in the formulation of clinical questions using PICO(T)** format (**PICO(T) = Patient population; Intervention or area of Interest; Comparison intervention or group; Outcome; Time).	O	O	O	O
Competency 4: Searches for external evidence*** to answer focused clinical questions (***external evidence = evidence generated from research).	O	O	O	O
Competency 5: Participates in critical appraisal of pre-appraised evidence**** (such as; clinical guidelines, evidence-based policies & procedures, and evidence summaries & syntheses).	O	O	O	O
Competency 6: Participates in critical appraisal of published research studies to determine their strength and applicability to clinical practice	O	O	O	O
Competency 7: Participates in the evaluation and synthesis of a body of evidence gathered to determine its' strength and applicability to clinical practice.	O	O	O	O
Competency 8: Collects practice data (e.g., individual patient data, quality improvement data) systematically as internal evidence for clinical decision making in the care of individuals, groups and populations.	O	O	O	O
Competency 9: Integrates evidence gathered from external and internal sources in order to plan evidence-based practice changes.	O	O	O	O
Competency 10: Implements practice changes based on evidence, clinical expertise and patient preferences to improve care processes and patient outcomes.	O	O	O	O
Competency 11: Evaluates outcomes of evidence-based decisions and practice changes for individuals, groups and populations to determine best practices.	O	O	O	O
Competency 12: Disseminates best practices supported by evidence to improve quality of care and patient outcomes.	O	O	O	O
Competency 13: Participates in strategies to sustain an evidence-based practice culture.	O	O	O	O

Figure 10.2   EBP competency self-assessment survey.

CREATING OPPORTUNITIES FOR INTERPROFESSIONAL LEARNING AND COLLABORATION

Evidence-based practice is a competency that is shared across all healthcare professional disciplines. The knowledge and skills needed to become proficient in evidence-based decision-making and care are the same regardless of discipline or specialty. The need to develop the shared competencies of EBP provides a unique opportunity for clinicians from across healthcare professions to learn and work together to develop knowledge and skills that are critical to their common goals of improving patient care and outcomes. In addition, these learning opportunities can stimulate interprofessional conversations, promote collaboration, and provide professionals with a chance to understand and value each other's experiences and perspectives.

Although the EBP competencies were developed through a Delphi study that included nurses only, the competencies have, nevertheless, been implemented in organizations across multiple disciplines with great success. (See Chapter 2 for a discussion on what a Delphi study entails.) When a shared understanding of EBP, usage of common language of EBP, and interprofessional participation in EBP become the standard approach to decision-making as well as the process that informs QI initiatives, best practice and quality care are the results.

DEVELOPING OTHER SKILLS

The EBP competencies can be used to measure not only EBP knowledge, skills, and attitudes but also other key attributes of nurses and other clinicians, including:

- **Technical skills:** Search for evidence via electronic databases and critically appraise literature using rapid critical appraisal (RCA) tools (see Chapter 5).

- **Critical thinking skills:** Identify important issues and articulate them clearly, integrate clinical expertise with evidence in decision-making, and consider patient and family preferences in decision-making.

- **Problem-solving skills:** Make recommendations for practice changes, adapt to changing situations/environments, and address barriers/resistance to change.

- **Communication skills:** Engage stakeholders, present outcomes of EBP practice change projects, and disseminate EBP work.

EXAMPLES OF INTEGRATION OF THE EBP COMPETENCIES

Healthcare systems in the United States have already begun to implement the new EBP competencies. For example, The Ohio State University Health System (Columbus, Ohio) has incorporated the EBP competencies into its job descriptions, clinical ladder system, and onboarding program while launching several other EBP initiatives. (Its progress is described in Chapter 11.) Nationwide Children's Hospital (Columbus, Ohio) has integrated the competencies into the working mechanisms of its policy and procedure committee. This transdisciplinary committee participated in a self-assessment on the EBP competencies, along with several other EBP initiatives, that provided data that informed the development of targeted education sessions for the group to increase their EBP knowledge and skills. In addition, ongoing mentoring has been provided to further develop and build their EBP skills. (Their progress is described in Chapter 12.)

SUMMARY

Evidence-based practice is an approach to decision-making and care that improves healthcare outcomes. Many organizations across the globe are implementing strategies to promote an EBP culture. Competence in EBP requires attainment of EBP knowledge, development of EBP skills, and an adoption of a positive attitude about EBP. The evidence-based practice competencies for practicing registered nurses and advanced practice nurses are a user-friendly tool that can rapidly facilitate implementation of evidence-based decision-making and care in an organization. By integrating the competencies into operational structures (mission statements, job descriptions, orientation programs, clinical ladders) and processes (policy and procedure committee work, shared governance council work, educational programs), an organization can begin to build a strong and effective EBP infrastructure or enhance an already existing EBP infrastructure.

REFERENCES

Aitken, L., & Patrician, P. (2000). Measuring organizational traits of hospitals: The Revised Nursing Work Index. *Nursing Research, 49*(3), 146–153.

American Nurses Association. (2000). *Nurse staffing and patient outcomes in the inpatient hospital setting.* Silver Spring, MD: American Nurses Association.

Covell, C. (2009). Outcomes achieved from organizational investment in nursing continuing professional development. *Journal of Nursing Administration, 39*(10), 438–443.

Dunn, S. V., Lawson, D., Robertson, S., Underwood, M., Clark, R., Valentine, T., & Herewane, D. (2000). The development of competency standards for specialist critical care nurses. *Journal of Advanced Nursing, 31*(2), 339–346.

Gallagher-Ford, L., Buck, J., & Melnyk, B. (2014). Leadership strategies and evidence-based practice competencies to sustain a culture and environment that supports best practice. In B. Melnyk & E. Fineout-Overholt (Eds.), *Evidence-based practice in nursing & healthcare: A guide to best practice* (3rd ed.), pp. xx–xx. Philadelphia, PA: Wolters Kluwer/Lippincott Williams & Wilkins.

Gellaty, I., Cowen, T., & Cummings, G. (2014). Staff nurses commitment, work relationships and turnover intention. *Nursing Research Online, 63*(3), 170–181.

Herscovitch, L., & Meyer, J. (2002). Commitment and organizational change: Extension of a three-component model. *Journal of Applied Psychology, 87*(3), 474–487.

Hughes, E. (2005). Nurses' perceptions of continuing professional development. *Nursing Standard, 19*(43), 50–54.

Ilic, D. (2009). Assessing competency in evidence based practice: Strengths and limitations of current tools in practice. *BioMed Central Medical Education, 9*(53). doi:10.1186/1472-6920-9-5

Joint Commission on Accreditation of Healthcare Organizations. (2002). *Healthcare at the crossroads: Strategies for addressing the evolving nursing crisis.* Washington, DC: Joint Commission.

Kramer, M., & Schmalenberg, C., (2004). Development and evaluation of essentials of magnetism tool. *Journal of Nursing Administration, 34*, 365–378.

Levett-Jones, T. (2005). Continuing education for nurses: A necessity or a nicety? *Continuing Education for Nurses, 36*(5), 229–233.

Liou, S. (2008). An analysis of the concept of organizational commitment. *Nursing Forum, 43*(3), 116–125.

Melnyk, B. M., Gallagher-Ford, L., Long, L. E., & Fineout-Overholt, E. (2014). The establishment of evidence-based practice competencies for practicing registered nurses and advanced practice nurses in real world clinical settings: Proficiencies to improve healthcare quality, reliability, patient outcomes, and costs. *Worldviews on Evidence-Based Nursing, 11*(1), 5–15.

Melnyk, B., Gallagher-Ford, L., & Troseth, M. (2016). Study of chief nurse executives indicates low prioritization of evidence-based practice and shortcomings in hospital performance metrics across the U.S. *Worldviews on Evidence-Based Nursing, 13*(1), 6–14. doi:10.1111/wvn.12133.

Meyer, J., Paunonen, S., Gellatly, I., Goffin, R., & Jackson, D. (1989). Organizational commitment and job performance: It's the nature of the commitment that counts. *Journal of Applied Psychology, 74*, 152–156.

Nolan, M., Owen, R., Curran, M., & Venables, A. (2000). Re-conceptualizing the outcomes of continuing professional development. *International Journal of Nursing Studies, 37*(October), 457–467.

Shamian, J. (1997). Towards quality and cost-effective health care. *International Nursing Review, 44*(3), 79–84.

Wilcock, P., Janes, G., & Chambers, A. (2009). Health care improvement and continuing interprofessional education: Continuing interprofessional development to improve patient outcomes. *Journal of Continuing Education in the Health Professions, 29*(2), 84–90. doi:10.1002

INTEGRATING THE EVIDENCE-BASED PRACTICE COMPETENCIES INTO THE ROLE OF ADVANCED PRACTICE NURSES

Jacalyn S. Buck, PhD, RN, NEA-BC; Sheila Chucta, MS, RN, CCRN, ACNS-BC; Deborah A. Francis, MS, BSN, RN-BC, ACNS-BC; Brenda K. Vermillion, DNP, RN, CCRN, ACNS-BC, ANP-BC; and Michele L. Weber, DNP, RN, CCRN, OCN, CCNS, APN-BC

KEY CONTENT IN THIS CHAPTER

- The "fit" for integrating EBP competencies into the clinical nurse specialist (CNS) role

- Successful strategies for integrating the EBP competencies into the CNS role

- Leveraging the CNS role to maximize EBP across the organization

- Return on investment (ROI) of the CNS as EBP mentor/champion across a large, complex organization

> If your actions inspire others to dream more, learn more, do more, and become more, you are a leader.
>
> *–John Quincy Adams*

Evidence-based practice (EBP) enhances healthcare by improving health outcomes, reducing costs, and improving the patient experience of care, including quality and satisfaction (Fineout-Overholt, Melnyk, & Schultz, 2005). It is estimated that EBP could improve patient outcomes by as much as 28% (Buntin et al., 2006). In 2009, the Institute of Medicine (IOM) recommended that 90% of clinical decisions be supported by practices reflecting the best available evidence by 2020. Yet, in the United States healthcare system, EBP is not consistently implemented or used (Stiffler & Cullen, 2010). In order to improve healthcare quality and patient outcomes, organizations must establish infrastructures to cultivate, implement, and sustain a culture that supports EBP.

The Advancing Research and Clinical practice through close Collaboration (ARCC) model is a conceptual framework that can be used to implement and sustain EBP across healthcare organizations (Melnyk & Fineout-Overholt, 2005). A key component of the ARCC model is the establishment of a cadre of ARCC EBP mentors who work with direct care providers to shift the culture from one of tradition, or "the way it has always been done," to one underpinned by EBP. Mentors also assist direct care providers with EBP projects and integrate EBP into daily practice to improve and sustain quality and patient care outcomes (Melnyk, 2007; Melnyk & Fineout-Overholt, 2015).

Key elements of the EBP mentor role include one-on-one mentoring, role-modeling, and working with staff to overcome barriers to EBP in an effort to transition to a practice environment where EBP thrives (Melnyk, 2007). Another critical role of EBP mentors is to stimulate and develop EBP knowledge and skills, otherwise known as *EBP competence*. Ultimately, these individuals strengthen direct care providers' beliefs about the importance of EBP *and* their ability to implement and sustain these practices (Melnyk & Fineout-Overholt, 2002). Clinical nurse specialists (CNS) are an excellent fit for the role of EBP mentor based on their educational preparation, clinical and practice expertise, influence at a micro- and macrosystem level, and ability to understand and lead EBP.

CLINICAL NURSE SPECIALISTS' ROLE IN EBP

The National Association of Clinical Nurse Specialists (NACNS) describes the role of the CNS as an advanced practice nurse (APN) with clinical expertise in diagnosis and treatment to prevent, remediate, or alleviate illness and promote health with a defined specialty population. The role of the CNS is to advance and promote professional nursing through EBP (NACNS, 2004). The CNS embodies the education, spheres of influence, competencies, and relationship with frontline nurses and interdisciplinary teams to be a key leader in EBP across healthcare organizations and systems.

The CNS is educationally prepared at the graduate level with a master's degree, doctorate in nursing practice (DNP) that focuses on EBP, or a doctorate of philosophy (PhD) with the focus on research. A recent survey of CNSs revealed that in addition to holding a master's degree, roughly 13% of the CNS respondents were educated at the doctoral level (NACNS, 2013). Advanced education enhances the CNS's ability to work collaboratively across disciplines to disseminate knowledge, implement best practice, and sustain change. Additionally, PhD prepared CNSs are educated to conduct research, lead research teams, and design and evaluate interventions for improved clinical and financial outcomes.

The focus for CNS practice is to achieve high-quality, efficient, cost-effective patient outcomes while translating research and EBP into clinical nursing care (Foster & Flanders, 2014; NACNS, 2004). These goals can be accomplished via improving clinical practice, developing appropriate use of current and new technologies, and creating new and innovative models of care. All these goals are enhanced when the CNS uses an EBP approach at the system level to create and implement improvements across the healthcare continuum for specialty groups of individuals, families, and communities (IOM, 2011; NACNS, 2012).

The five domains of CNS practice reflect the flexibility and diversity of the CNS role and include consultation, leadership, research, clinical practice, and education (Heitkemper & Bond, 2004). Within the five domains of practice are three interrelated and overlapping spheres of influence: the patient, the nurse, and the system (NACNS, 2004). It is within and across these five domains and three spheres that the CNS influences, facilitates, and implements EBP. The description of the variety and breadth of the CNS role reflects how well the CNS is positioned to excel as an EBP leader and mentor across the healthcare continuum.

Sphere of Influence: The Patient

The CNS has direct interaction with patients, families, and populations to promote health and well-being and to improve quality of life by using a holistic approach in the advanced nursing management of health, illness, and disease states (NACNS, 2010). The CNS contributes to patient outcomes by:

- Assisting staff in the development of innovative, cost-effective programs or protocols of care

- Providing leadership for collaborative, evidence-based plans of care

- Identifying when evidence-based guidelines, policies, procedures, and/or plans of care need to be tailored to the individual, family, or population

Sphere of Influence: The Nurse

The CNS works with frontline nurses through collaboration and influence to continuously improve patient outcomes and promote environments of clinical excellence through implementation of evidence-based nursing care standards and programs of care (Foster & Flanders, 2014; Hanson, 2015; NACNS, 2004). Gallagher-Ford (2012) and Gerrish et al. (2012) identified factors that influence an advanced practice nurse's (APN) ability to promote EBP among frontline staff nurses. These influencing factors include personal attributes, knowledge and skill in EBP, clinical credibility with frontline staff, and leadership style.

These findings support the role of the CNS as an EBP leader and mentor with frontline nursing staff. Their expertise in nursing practice aids to advance the care of patients and families and improve clinical outcomes. The range and diversity of the CNS role is reflected in the fact that they provide guidance and education at both the micro- and macrosystem level while still spending a significant portion of their time providing direct patient care, consulting with nursing staff and others, teaching nurses and other staff, and leading and assisting with EBP projects (NACNS, 2012).

Sphere of Influence: The System

Providing system-level leadership along with change management is a crucial element of the CNS role. These individuals use change theories/management to promote adoption of EBP and innovations in care delivery. Additionally, the CNS facilitates the provision of clinically competent care through education, role-modeling, team-building, and quality monitoring. CNSs specify expected clinical- and system-level outcomes by designing programs to improve clinical and system-level processes (NACNS, 2010).

THE CNS AS AN EBP MENTOR

Although progress is being made, EBP remains challenging for frontline staff. Barriers to using and sustaining EBP that have been identified by frontline staff include inadequate knowledge and skills, lack of time, and lack of support (Gerrish et al., 2011a; Melnyk et al., 2004). Clinical nurse specialists can be critical players in addressing these EBP barriers and advancing EBP among frontline nurses in their ability to engage, influence, and assist staff members and use the knowledge and skills required for EBP. They can serve as mentors, educators, change agents, and translators of research for the frontline staff (Gerrish et al., 2011b, 2012; Melnyk, Gallagher-Ford, Long, & Fineout-Overholt, 2014; Smith, Donzo, Cole, Johnston, & Giebe, 2009).

Evidence-based CNSs are especially well suited to advance EBP in that they also hold the knowledge, skills, and experience to fulfill the seven roles that a mentor provides to mentees: teacher, sponsor, advisor, agent, role model, coach, and confidant (Smith et al., 2009; Tobin, 2004). Mentoring others in EBP is an important factor, not only in implementing EBP in an organization, but especially in sustaining EBP over time. Because of their unique blend of proficiencies, it is logical to recognize that CNSs are excellent candidates to be educated and empowered to assume the role and responsibilities of EBP mentors for healthcare organizations.

THE CNS AND THE EBP COMPETENCIES

In 2014, Melnyk and colleagues published their work on the establishment of EBP competencies for the registered nurse and the APN. The authors listed 13 EBP competencies for registered nurses (RNs) with an additional 11 for APNs (see Chapter 2 for a list). All the advanced practice EBP competencies align beautifully with the stated intent and scope of the CNS; therefore, the CNS role is an optimal APN role for integration of the EBP competencies. The EBP competencies that focus on research are those that center on searching and evaluating the healthcare literature and implementing research findings into practice.

The CNS is tied to the clinical environment and sees the challenges that frontline staff face on a daily basis. The CNS is immersed in the clinical practice of a specialty area, and as the master clinician, the CNS is aware of what has been published in the healthcare literature within his or her scope of clinical practice. The CNS has the skill set to evaluate the current body of literature to determine whether there is sufficient evidence to support a practice change or whether more research needs to be conducted.

Because of this strong link to clinical practice, the CNS is able to assist with the decision-making when evidence-based clinical practices need to be implemented. CNSs also are able to lead EBP changes successfully due to their foundational skills in leading interdisciplinary teams, measuring processes and outcomes, and formulating evidence-based policies and procedures. In addition, CNSs' conceptual understanding of the healthcare microsystem and macrosystem allows them to see the need and implement clinical practices at a unit, department, or health-system level. Following a clinical practice change, the CNS provides clinical support, leadership, and education, which are all essential skills and tactics to sustain the change.

Finally, the CNS assists in developing the evidence-based clinical culture of the unit or department. CNSs can role-model translation of research findings into daily practice in many ways; for example, they use findings published in the educational literature regarding adult learning principles and use of simulation to design classes for new frontline staff. They also use research information regarding effective approaches to leading and mentoring staff at different levels of experience (newer staff need different support than more seasoned staff). The CNS can encourage and assist frontline staff to think critically about clinical issues and problems while mentoring them in unique ways to use an evidence-based approach to improve the situation.

Some issues that arise on the clinical units are related to communication, and impaired communication can inhibit patients from receiving excellent care from all members of the healthcare team. The CNS can use current evidence related to communication and translate that information/knowledge into actions to improve communication among members of the interprofessional care team. These examples of translation of research from across disciplines demonstrate the wide variety of opportunities the CNS has to role-model and implement an evidence-based approach to care that promotes improvement in practices and outcomes.

BUILDING THE INFRASTRUCTURE FOR EBP AT AN ACADEMIC MEDICAL CENTER THROUGH THE ROLE OF THE CNS

The development and implementation of the EBP mentor role as part of the CNS role is a pivotal undertaking in any organization. The research-based EBP competencies are valuable tools in any ongoing work to build an infrastructure that underpins the EBP culture and environment. In this section, we outline the journey that one hospital undertook—The Ohio State University Wexner Medical Center (OSUWMC)—to integrate EBP into its culture.

The EBP journey began in 2011, with the partnership with the Center for Trans-disciplinary Evidence-based Practice (CTEP) at The Ohio State University College of Nursing to integrate EBP in the nursing enterprise. Together, they built the EBP infrastructure and developed EBP knowledge and skills in the organization with great success.

Realignment of CNS in the Organizational Structure

One of the key activities in this journey has been the sound integration of EBP into the role of the CNS in a variety of ways throughout the organization. Some of the critical steps undertaken by nursing administration at the University Hospital (UH) and Ross Heart Hospital (RHH) to advance nursing practice through application of best evidence and to build a culture of inquiry included:

- The CNSs in UH and RHH attended an intensive 5-day EBP education and skills-building program. This program provided the CNSs with a "deep dive" immersion into the steps of EBP process, how to manage change, and how to mentor others.

- All CNSs were realigned to report to the Health System Nursing Quality, Research, EBP, and Education Department. This realignment created an overarching structure that promoted the translation of evidence into bedside practice and aligned that work with quality initiatives at the unit level to improve clinical outcomes.

These early changes set the stage for the integration of the EBP competencies, which served as the next step in "hard-wiring" EBP into the CNS role and their performance expectations.

CNS EBP Competency Advancement

EBP is interwoven with the five domains of CNS practice; therefore, understanding EBP is essential to the CNS role. Nursing leaders within the OSUWMC Health System collaborated with the CTEP at the College of Nursing in an effort to advance EBP skill development for the CNS team and create a cadre of ARCC

EBP mentors. The goal of this collaboration was to establish a consistent and standardized educational venue regarding the EBP process and mentor role, as well as to allow the CNSs to actualize within their role in the organization.

All practicing in the CNS role were encouraged and supported to attend a 5-day EBP immersion course at The Ohio State University College of Nursing. The program provided a deep dive into the concept and process of EBP. Included in the course were successful strategies for developing a culture of inquiry and implementing and sustaining EBP within an organization. As part of the course, participants received actual experience through expert mentoring in developing a structured clinical question executing an appropriate search for evidence, developing an action plan for implementing EBP changes, and integrating EBP into their organizational culture. Attending this immersion established the expectation for the CNS to embrace the EBP competency, "systematically conducts an exhaustive search for external evidence to answer clinical questions" (Melnyk et al., 2014, p. 7)

Many of the clinical questions posed by the CNSs in this course revealed sound evidence leading to the implementation of practice changes within the organization. Examples of this include:

- Support with implementation of the Modified Early Warning Score (MEWS) tool into the electronic health record (EHR), followed by usage in clinical practice to assist with early recognition of a decompensating patient.

- Implementation of a program to decrease the frequency of vital signs at night in stable patients in an effort to improve a patient's ability to sleep, heal, and recover.

- Implementation of a new suctioning protocol order set for new tracheostomy patients based on need rather than standard times.

In addition to improving their EBP competencies as well as gaining EBP mentor status, several CNSs have become CTEP-EBP facilitators. This supplementary EBP mentoring experience, along with a library of resources and information databases for the acquisition and appraisal of best evidence sources, enables

CNSs to support, advocate, and mentor EBP at the unit, department, and system level. The CNSs serve as EBP mentors and demonstrate competency in EBP and change implementation to improve patient outcomes on a consistent basis.

Integration of the Newly Published EBP Competencies

Upon publication of the EBP competences for RNs and APNs, the decision was made to integrate the competencies into the CNS role and job descriptions.

Onboarding: Orientation to the CNS Role in the Organization

The introduction to EBP begins during the hiring and orientation process for all nurses in the organization. It is expected that CNSs, as APNs, demonstrate the core CNS competencies as well as the APN EBP competencies (see Chapter 2) within their clinical domains of practice. The CNS is responsible for providing and facilitating the provision of direct and indirect care for patients and families. Capable of managing complex, unpredictable patient care situations, the CNS provides consultation and collaboration with all members of the healthcare team. They serve as a role model and resource for frontline staff within the unit, department, health system, and the community.

Position Description

The CNS position description in the organization describes the role of the CNS within the healthcare system. It provides insight on expectation of the role but allows for autonomy in order for the CNS to meet the needs and generate positive outcomes for the patient, staff, and health system. The position description allows the CNS to capitalize on his/her unique skills and style of interaction.

The position description for the CNS has always embodied the five domains of the CNS practice; however, now the position description also embodies the APN EBP competencies (Heitkemper & Bond, 2004; Melnyk et al., 2014):

- **Clinical practice and leadership domains:** The CNS continuously evaluates the gaps between current nursing practice and evidence-based nursing practice and implements best practice initiatives when appropriate. CNSs may develop, review, revise, and interpret patient care standards or nursing clinical practice guidelines related to their area of clinical specialty. These standards and guidelines are often the basis of care at the bedside and use the CNS's advance practice skill of conducting an exhaustive search of the literature to ensure practice is based on the best evidence. As a leader, the CNS must demonstrate best practices and provide the rationale regarding why these standards are important in patient care. Additionally, the CNS is often directly involved in implementing and evaluating new techniques and equipment for safety. An essential leadership skill for the CNS is change facilitation and management. The CNS must be able to implement and sustain change initiatives of varying complexity at the microsystem and/or macrosystem level.

- **Research domain:** The CNS uses EBP to assist in program planning to improve patient outcomes, services, operations, and cost. It is anticipated that the CNS critically appraises nursing research, disseminates the findings, and implements change as appropriate. The CNS also collaborates with the nurse scientist on research projects when evidence to answer a question is found to be insufficient.

- **Education:** The CNS supports frontline nursing staff development through mentoring, consultation, educational presentations, and clinical direction. The CNS is often asked to serve as an EBP mentor for staff to assist them in developing projects at the bedside. These frontline nursing staff range from new hires in a nurse residency role to experienced staff that have applied for and been accepted into nurse fellowship programs, or nurses applying for the career ladder program. This is an exciting part of the CNS role because staff members identify an area of interest and begin the EBP process to identify a project that can impact the care that they deliver at the bedside. Mentoring staff in the EBP process is a strategy that can help sustain a culture of EBP.

- **Consultation:** The CNS provides expertise on committees in addition to collaborating with peers and interprofessional team members. In this role, the CNS can lead "transdisciplinary teams in applying synthesized evidence to initiate clinical decisions and practice changes to improve the health of indi-viduals, groups, and populations" (Melnyk et al., 2014, p. 7). It is crucial that in this consultative role, the CNS assists in development of the evidence but also reviews interventions that the frontline staff may be required to provide. In the consultative role, the CNS must assure that the interventions are achievable within the clinical setting so that frontline staff are not resis-tant to proposed practice change, thereby assuring success of the project.

The CNS role is multifaceted, as evidenced by the five domains of practice. How-ever, introduction of APN EBP competencies into the CNS job description has provided a foundation for clinical practice. A job description that embodies the domains of practice and the EBP competencies has served as a practice catalyst for both the novice and experienced CNS. It has also provided a structure and process for EBP projects and assisted in measurement of individual professional growth and development, as well as for annual accomplishments.

Nurse Residency Program

Throughout the organization, new graduate nurses participate in a 12-month nurse residency professional development program, in which the nurses engage in an EBP group project where the CNSs serve as EBP mentors for these new nurses, supporting and encouraging them through the EBP process, from clinical inquiry through project dissemination. Topics such as staffing and assignment patterns, quality issues such as falls and infection prevention, and factors related to staff satisfaction have all been highlighted. The time spent working together on these projects has promoted an ongoing mentoring relationship between the CNSs and these new nurses.

Shared Governance Councils

The CNSs are active participants and represented in all the organizational shared governance councils, with many serving as chairpersons and co-chairpersons. These councils provide a forum for discussion and shared decision-making, where nurses build on their collective expertise to develop, implement, evaluate, and modify nursing practice across the healthcare system. CNSs function as EBP mentors throughout the shared governance structure by assuring that the best evidence is consistently used to solve clinical issues and concerns brought forward to the councils. The shared governance councils within the healthcare system include:

- **Patient Care Council:** Oversees the development and approval process for clinical standards; coordinates and facilitates nursing quality initiatives and the use of evidence-based practice and research to improve patient care delivery and outcomes.

- **Professional Development Council:** Provides strategic direction, consultation, and recommendations for educational programs to meet the educational and professional development needs of nurses throughout the healthcare system.

- **Research, EBP, and Innovation Council:** Fosters the development of nursing research and EBP priorities by facilitating and advising nurses in the development, application, publication, and presentation of nursing research, EBP, and other scholarly activities.

- **Unit Collaboration Council:** Establishes a mechanism of communication between nursing units and the shared governance councils; provides a forum for health system Unit Leadership Councils (ULC) chairs to discuss goals and objectives of business units and other professional nursing and patient care issues; promotes nursing excellence by providing guidance for nursing recognition, recruitment, and retention.

- **Coordinating Council:** Facilitates communication and coordination across the decision-making bodies of the four health system councils and ULCs; functions to integrate efforts of the health system councils; assists with information sharing; encourages efficiency in resolving issues regarding nursing practice; supports nursing goals.

Additionally, several subcouncils have been created out of the shared governance research council. The Fall Practice Problem Group (FPPG) and the Wound Practice Problem Group (WPPG) are working councils that address priorities for optimal safe and quality patient care in the practice environment. All subcouncils are both led and facilitated by a CNS who is also an EBP mentor.

Evidence-based practice is consistently used to translate new knowledge related to patient falls, falls with injury, and wound prevention. For example, the ongoing mission of the FPPG is to explore, evaluate, and disseminate the current evidence to advance nursing's knowledge of factors contributing to patient falls, fall risk-factor assessments, fall-prevention interventions, and fall injury-reduction strategies. These group processes include:

- Reviewing current unit, department, and business unit falls data to identify trends

- Critically evaluating the literature to identify best practices in fall risk-factor assessment, fall prevention, and injury reduction

- Systematically reviewing and assembling internal and external resources and tools for fall data reporting and analysis, falls assessment, fall prevention, and injury reduction

- Reviewing relevant nursing policies and procedures, identifying disparities between current practice and best practice in fall prevention and injury reduction, and recommending, as appropriate, revisions to nursing standards of practice to integrate best practices

- Providing consultation to individuals, units, and teams seeking expert guidance

- Identifying potential quality improvement, EBP, and research opportunities for development and implementation

- Disseminating the compilation of knowledge and tools through the channels of collaboration, consultation, and circulation of best practices

- Serving as champions of EBP and nursing innovations in patient safety and fall prevention/injury reduction

The Fall Risk Stratification Wheel (the "wheel") provides an example of an outcome from this group; see Figure 11.1.

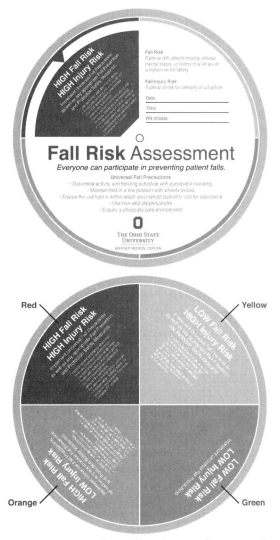

Figure 11.1   The Fall Risk Stratification Wheel.

The wheel, which serves as a visual communication tool for all staff, family, and visitors, is placed in the patient's room or on his or her door to convey the patient's current risk for falling and risk for injury if a fall occurs (Hefner, McAlearney, Mansfield, Knupp, & Moffatt-Bruce, 2015). Additionally, the FPPG created a post-fall huddle tool and maintains the Falls Resource page on the organizational intranet.

Using the most current and updated evidence, the WPPG developed a Wound Product Guide. This resource is available to all staff and includes a comprehensive list of wound care products, their classification, product points, indications for use, cautions for use, contraindications, sizing choices, application and removal directions, and dressing change recommendations. This guide resides on the Skin/Wound Care Management Resource site that is located on the organization's intranet. This site was developed and is maintained by the WPPG. Additionally, the group provides innovative solutions to improve and enhance the wound documentation within the EHR.

Clinical Ladder Program

The organizational career ladder program, Clinical Ladder program, recognizes and rewards staff nurses for their clinical expertise in delivering direct care to patients. Frontline staff nurses are acknowledged and promoted with this designation through demonstration of expertise in areas of clinical management, educational activities, EBP, and research. Many CNSs have achieved Clinical Ladder status as frontline nurses and now, as EBP mentors, assist other frontline nurses through this process.

Standards of Nursing Practice

The Clinical Standards and Practice Committee provide a review of the nursing policies and procedures for OSUWMC. The CNSs serve as EBP mentors on this committee by reviewing the current and relevant evidence, critically appraising the evidence, and integrating new evidence into the policies and procedures. Evidence tables are created and used to assist with this process and document this ongoing work. Clinical nurse specialists also employ a similar process to assist with the creation of new policies and clinical practice guidelines within the organization.

Clinical Practice, Quality and Patient Safety

At the unit and department level, the CNSs participate on quality improvement (QI) committees where they mentor frontline staff nurses from their respective areas through continually evaluating and improving the quality of care provided. When areas for improvement are identified, steps are taken to review current literature and implement EBP when appropriate.

Staff Education and Professional Development

Clinical nurse specialists use evidence to develop and update the tools used throughout the onboarding process. These tools are used to track and document new staff progression, evaluate preceptor feedback, and provide clinical expertise and guidance. This process continues as CNSs incorporate EBP into the frontline staff annual competencies. An example of this process can be highlighted through the integration of simulation technology into the medical surgical nurse competency assessments to enhance nurses' competencies. In this example, a strong body of nursing literature revealed that "failure to rescue" was a quality issue identified in inpatient environments across the United States (AHRQ, 2005; Ashcraft, 2004; Dillon, Noble, & Kaplan, 2009; Duff, Gardiner, & Barnes, 2007; Friese & Aiken, 2008; Moldenhauer, Sabel, Chu, & Mehler, 2009; NQF, 2004; Shapiro et al., 2004; Wilson, Burke, Priest, & Salas, 2005). In a proactive attempt to avoid this issue, the CNS team in the medical surgical area developed a simulation program to assess nurses' abilities to recognize and respond to scenarios involving decompensating patients and to provide education during the scenarios.

Clinical nurse specialists are involved in clinical initiatives throughout the organization and consistently use and refine their EBP competencies and EBP mentor skills. Examples include:

- Providing input and clinical expertise in creating and sustaining the first organizational innovation unit

- Creating and implementing of a new nursing role (Clinical Coordinator) and model of care to improve care coordination and transition of care

- Continuing investigation and follow-up with unit- and department-specific clinical and quality issues and participation in issue-specific task forces

- Working in synergy with the clinical nurse scientist by contributing, collaborating, and participating in nursing research

SUMMARY

In the era of healthcare reform, it is important for leaders to identify individuals who can influence and shape practice steeped in evidence to deliver high-quality patient outcomes. The ARCC model provides an organizational framework for implementing and sustaining evidence-based practice with evidence-based practice mentors as a central component. Because the focus of the CNS role is to achieve high-quality, efficient, cost-effective patient outcomes while translating research and EBP into clinical nursing care, the CNS as the EBP mentor is a perfect fit. Integrating EBP mentor responsibilities into the CNS role has been an effective strategy to build and sustain a culture of EBP across the healthcare organization.

REFERENCES

Agency for Healthcare Research and Quality (AHRQ). (2005). 2005 National Healthcare Quality Report. Retrieved from http://archive.ahrq.gov/qual/nhqr05/nhqr05.pdf

Ashcraft, A. (2004). Differentiating between pre-arrest and failure-to-rescue. *MEDSURG Nursing, 13*(4), 211–215.

Buntin, M., Damberg, C., Haviland, A., Kapur, K., Lurie, N., McDevitt, R., & Marquis, M. S. (2006). Consumer-directed health care: Early evidence about effects on cost and quality. *Health Affairs, 25*(6), W516–W530.

Dillon, P., Noble, K., & Kaplan, L. (2009). Simulation as a means to foster collaborative interdisciplinary education. *Nursing Education Perspectives, 30*(2), 87–90.

Duff, B., Gardiner, G., & Barnes, M. (2007). The impact of surgical ward nurses practicing respiratory assessment on positive patient outcomes. *Australian Journal of Advanced Nursing, 24*(4), 52–56.

Fineout-Overholt, E., Melnyk, B., & Schultz, A. (2005). Transforming health care from the inside out: Advancing evidence-based practice in the 21st century. *Journal of Professional Nursing, 21*(6), 335–344.

Foster, J., and Flanders, S. (2014). Challenges in CNS practice and education. *The Online Journal of Issues in Nursing, 19*(2). Retrieved from http://www.nursingworld.org/MainMenuCategories/ANAMarketplace/ANA-Periodicals/OJIN/TableofContents/Vol-19-2014/No2-May-2014/Challenges-in-CNS-Education-and-Practice.html

Friese, C. R., & Aiken, L. H. (2008). Failure to rescue in the surgical oncology population: Implications for nursing and quality improvement. *Oncology Nursing Forum, 35*(5), 779–785.

Gallagher-Ford, L. (2012). Advanced practice nurses using role modeling, teaching, clinical problem solving, and change facilitation to promote evidence-based practice among clinical staff nurses: Commentary. (2), 55–56. doi:10.1136/ebnurs

Gerrish, K., Guillaume, L., Kirshbaum, M., McDonnell, A., Tod, A., & Nolan, M. (2011a). Factors influencing the contribution of advanced practice nurses to promoting evidence-based practice among front-line nurses: Findings from a cross-sectional study. *Journal of Advanced Nursing, 67*(5), 1079–1090.

Gerrish, K., McDonnell, A., Nolan, M., Guillaume, L., Kirschbaum, L., & Tod, A. (2011b). The role of advanced practice nurses in knowledge brokering as a means of promoting evidence-based practice among clinical nurses. *Journal of Advanced Nursing, 67*(9), 2004–2014. doi:10.1111/j.1365-2648.2011.05642.x

Gerrish, K., Nolan, M., McDonnell, A., Tod, A., Kirshbaum, M., & Guillaume, G. (2012). Factors influencing advanced practice nurses' ability to promote evidence-based practice among frontline nurses. *Worldviews on Evidence-Based Nursing, 9*(1), 30–39.

Hanson, D. M. (2015). Role of the clinical nurse specialist in the journey to magnet recognition. *AACN Advanced Critical Care, 26*(1), 50–57.

Hefner, J. L., McAlearney, A. S., Mansfield, J., Knupp, A. M., & Moffatt-Bruce, S. D. (2015). A falls wheel in a large academic medical center: An intervention to reduce patient falls with harm. *Journal for Healthcare Quality, 37*(6), 374–380.

Heitkemper, M., & Bond, E. (2004). Clinical nurse specialists: State of the profession and challenges ahead. *Clinical Nurse Specialist, 18*(3), 135–240.

Institute of Medicine (IOM; U.S.) Roundtable on Evidence-Based Medicine. (2009). *Leadership commitments to improve value in healthcare: Finding common ground: Workshop summary.* Washington, DC: National Academies Press. Retrieved from http://www.ncbi.nlm.nih.gov/books/NBK52847/

Institute of Medicine (IOM). (2011). *The future of nursing: Leading change, advancing health.* Washington, DC: National Academies Press. Retrieved from http://www.thefutureofnursing.org/sites/default/files/Future%20of%20Nursing%20Report_0.pdf

Melnyk, B. M. (2007). The evidence-based practice mentor: A promising strategy for implementing and sustaining EBP in healthcare systems. *Worldviews on Evidence-Based Nursing, 4*(3), 123–125.

Melnyk, B. M., & Fineout-Overholt, E. (2002). Putting research into practice. *Reflections on Nursing Leadership, 28*(2), 22–25.

Melnyk, B., & Fineout-Overholt, E. (2005). *ARCC advancing research and clinical practice through close collaboration.* Gilbert, AZ: ARCC Publishing.

Melnyk, B. M., & Fineout-Overholt, E. (2015). *Evidence-based practice in nursing & healthcare: A guide to best practice* (3rd ed.). Philadelphia, PA: Wolters Kluwer.

Melnyk, B. M., Fineout-Overholt, E., Fischbeck Feinstein, N., Li, H., Small, L., Wilcox, L., & Kraus, R. (2004). Nurses' perceived knowledge, beliefs, skills and needs regarding evidence-based practice: Implications for accelerating the paradigm shift. *Worldviews on Evidence-Based Nursing, 1*(3), 185–193.

Melnyk, B. M., Gallagher-Ford, L., Long, L. E., & Fineout-Overholt, E. (2014). The establishment of evidence-based practice competencies for practicing registered nurses and advanced practice nurses in real-world clinical settings: Proficiencies to improve healthcare quality, reliability, patient outcomes and costs. *Worldviews on Evidence-Based Nursing, 11*(1), 5–15.

Moldenhauer, K., Sabel, A., Chu, E. S., & Mehler, P. S. (2009). Clinical triggers: An alternative to a rapid response team. *The Joint Commission Journal on Quality and Patient Safety, 35*(3), 164–174.

National Association of Clinical Nurse Specialists (NACNS). (2004). *Statement on clinical nurse specialist practice and education* (2nd ed.). Retrieved from http://www.nacns.org/docs/NACNS-Statement.pdf

National Association of Clinical Nurse Specialists (NACNS). (2010). Executive summary 2006–2008, The CNS Competency Task Force. Retrieved from http://www.nacns.org/docs/CNSCoreCompetenciesBroch.pdf

National Association of Clinical Nurse Specialists (NACNS). (2012). The National Association of Clinical Nurse Specialists (NACNS) response to the Institute of Medicine's Future of Nursing report. Retrieved from http://www.nacns.org/docs/IOM-Recommendations1203.pdf

National Association of Clinical Nurse Specialists (NACNS). (2013). CNS FAQs. Retrieved from http://www.nacns.org/html/cns-faqs.php

National Quality Forum (NQF). (2004). National voluntary consensus standards for nursing-sensitive care. An initial performance measure set. Retrieved from https://www.qualityforum.org/Projects/n-r/Nursing-Sensitive_Care_Initial_Measures/Nursing_Sensitive_Care__Initial_Measures.aspx

Shapiro, M., Morey, J., Small, S., Langford, V., Kaylor, C., Jagminas, L., ... Jay, G. (2004). Simulation based teamwork training for emergency staff: Does it improve clinical team performance when added to an existing didactic teamwork curriculum? *Quality & Safety in Health Care, 13*, 417–421.

Smith, J., Donze, A., Cole, F., Johnston, J., & Giebe, J. (2009). Neonatal advanced practice nurses as key facilitators in implementing evidence-based practice. *Neonatal Network, 28*(3), 193–201.

Stiffler, D., & Cullen, D. (2010). Evidence-based practice for nurse practitioner students: A competency-based teaching framework. *Journal of Professional Nursing, 26*(5), 272–277.

Tobin, C. (2004). Mentoring: Seven roles and some specifics. *American Journal of Respiratory Critical Care, 170*(2), 114–117.

Wilson, K. A., Burke, C. S., Priest, H. A., & Salas, E. (2005). Promoting health care safety through training high reliability teams. *Quality & Safety in Health Care, 14*(4), 303–309.

CHAPTER 12

USING THE EVIDENCE-BASED PRACTICE COMPETENCIES WITH POLICY AND PROCEDURE COMMITTEES

Cheryl Boyd, PhD, RN, NE-BC, WHNP-BC, CNS, and Julie Gerberick, MS, RN, CEN

KEY CONTENT IN THIS CHAPTER

- EBP competencies can be integrated into healthcare organizations in innovative ways

- Integration of the EBP competencies across a multidisciplinary team builds EBP knowledge and skills

- Integration of the EBP competencies in a policy and procedure review committee promotes a culture of evidence-based practice in an organization

> "Teamwork is the ability to work together toward a common vision. The ability to direct individual accomplishments toward organizational objectives. It is the fuel that allows common people to attain uncommon results."
>
> –Andrew Carnegie

Nationwide Children's Hospital (NCH), located in Columbus, Ohio, is a 464-bed pediatric, tertiary care, three-time Magnet®-designated hospital. Nationally ranked as one of the *U.S. News & World Report* America's Best Children's Hospitals, NCH has a reputation for providing excellence in patient care. The NCH strategic plan guides the journey to best outcomes through the best people and programs. The organization believes that values such as teamwork, respect, innovation, and safety lead to best patient outcomes. Evidence-based practice (EBP) is recognized at NCH as an effective approach to care that contributes to improved health, reduced costs, and decreased patient morbidity. Clinical decisions based on the systematic search, critical appraisal, and synthesis of research, along with internal evidence from quality improvement or management projects, support high-quality clinical decisions (Melnyk & Fineout-Overholt, 2011).

EBP COMPETENCY AND THE PATIENT/ FAMILY CARE POLICY COMMITTEE

Patient care practices and procedures used by NCH nurses, respiratory therapists, pharmacists, social workers, and other disciplines are managed by the Patient/ Family Care Policy Committee. Committee membership includes 26 members who represent staff and leadership and a chairperson. The committee's chairperson is an experienced nurse practitioner (NP) who is currently the Director of Professional Development and the hospital's Magnet® Program Director. The organization values interprofessional collaboration and for many years has staffed the committee with representatives from across disciplines, representing a variety of clinical settings and positions. The committee members are selected for their experience and expertise. Table 12.1 lists work settings and positions.

TABLE 12.1 NATIONWIDE CHILDREN'S HOSPITAL PATIENT/FAMILY CARE COMMITTEE

Positions Represented	Departments Represented
Clinical Vice President	Patient Care Services Administration
Director	Pharmacy
Nurse Supervisor	Laboratory Services
Assistant Nurse Manager	Quality Improvement Services
Respiratory Care Manager	Ambulatory Services
Pharmacy Manager	Legal Services
Epidemiology Specialist	Nursing Research
Education Specialists: Central and Unit-based	Epidemiology
Advanced Practice Registered Nurse	Emergency Services
Nurse Scientist	Medical-Surgical Nursing
Staff Nurse	Critical Care Nursing
	Neonatal Services
	Perioperative Services
	Social Work
	Urgent Care
	Risk Management
	Pain Team
	Respiratory Therapy
	Advanced Practice Registered Nursing
	Professional Development
	Homecare

The committee is responsible for updating and developing practice policies that are evidence-based. The policies and procedures are the major clinical practice resource that staff access to guide clinical practice.

Although the members are responsible to lead teams outside the committee in the development and review of policies and procedures, the chairperson recognized that the members' EBP knowledge and skills (competencies) had never been assessed or addressed. The committee members generally felt they were reviewing policies and procedures and implementing practice changes based on evidence. However, taking time to locate evidence had been a challenge, and sometimes the teams overlooked important stakeholders' clinical practice preferences. Articles related to the policies being reviewed were discussed in committee, and lists of references were often made available for committee members and staff to review. However, questions often arose about the possibility of improving skills in literature searching, locating national standards of practice, and evaluating the quality of the research, standards, and best practices that were being reviewed.

As a Magnet® organization, applying research and EBP to practice is required (American Nurses Credentialing Center, 2013), yet enculturating those processes into daily practice is challenging. Findings in a 2012 study (Melnyk, Fineout-Overholt, Gallagher-Ford, & Kaplan) indicated that even in Magnet organizations, nurses felt they needed even more knowledge and skills in EBP. Having enough time to adequately review evidence and the skills to critically appraise the literature were reported as barriers by the committees, and members reported that EBP was not taught in their healthcare programs.

A COST-EFFECTIVE EBP COMPETENCY ASSESSMENT AND EDUCATION

Many EBP studies focus on the clinical care of providers at the bedside, yet few have focused on the infrastructure of a policy committee and its contribution to an EBP organizational culture (Melnyk & Gallagher-Ford, 2014). To support the organizational culture necessary to deliver high-quality evidence-based care, the chair of the Patient/Family Policy Committee approached the committee with the idea to put a plan into place for improved EBP competency. All members agreed that they were interested in EBP skill development. If the NCH policy committee was to align itself with the Institute of Medicine (IOM) 2020 goal that 90% of clinical decisions be evidence-based, then positioning the committee for improved EBP practice should lead to better patient outcomes (Melnyk & Fineout-Overholt, 2015; Melnyk et al., 2012). Accomplishing an interprofessional improvement project with such a large, diverse committee was challenging.

The hospital has clinical placement agreements with many college and university nursing programs, including The Ohio State University College of Nursing, to provide high-quality clinical experiences and nurse preceptors for undergraduate and graduate nursing students. That partnership was the underpinning that evolved into an EBP collaboration. The director reached out and partnered with an EBP expert consultant/faculty from The Ohio State University College of Nursing to develop a practical, cost-effective approach to providing EBP education and skills-building. The chair invited the consultant to meet the committee.

An EBP self-report competency survey was administered to the policy committee to determine EBP baseline knowledge, as well as their beliefs about the EBP knowledge and skill of their expert teams. The survey was based on the EBP competencies (Melnyk, Gallagher-Ford, Long, & Fineout-Overholt, 2014). Electronic survey questions were sent to the committee with a timeline for response. Participation reminders were also sent to the committee.

Fifty-three percent of the committee participated. The results of the survey were presented the next time the consultant visited the committee. The committee rated themselves between a 2 (indicating needs improvement) and a 3 (indicating some competence) on a 5-point scale for each EBP competency. An education plan for the committee was developed based on the survey results.

DETERMINING AN INTERPROFESSIONAL EDUCATION FRAMEWORK

Although educational collaboration between nurses and other healthcare disciplines is not typical in most organizations, interprofessional collaboration can be improved by educating doctors, nurses, and other health professionals and also by assisting providers to work together (Robert Wood Johnson Foundation,

2011). Therefore, the chair, committee, and consultant collectively decided that the education plan would include sessions when the committee was together. The educational framework for the EBP education was an interprofessional process built upon recommendations and competencies from the IOM. To respond appropriately to complex patient needs and deliver high-quality evidenced-based care, the IOM directed professionals to work collaboratively, rather than in parallel. In 2003, the IOM defined five core competencies that all healthcare professional education should meet (IOM, 2003). Three of those competencies directly pertained to the committee's project:

- Provide patient-centered care

- Work in interdisciplinary teams

- Employ evidence-based practice

Working in interprofessional teams and collaboration are new concepts that are not easy to grasp given that these professionals have been educated in separate programs that operate in their respective silos. Additional concepts that supported the program were based upon a published report from the Interprofessional Education Collaborative Expert Panel (2011) that described the interrelationships among the IOM core competencies and framed the interprofessional focus. For example, the provision of patient-centered care (the first competency) is the objective of interprofessional teamwork (the second competency). The relationship between the patient and the healthcare team defines the work of the interprofessional team. Another core competency—evidence-based practice—informs the team about appropriate patient care processes.

The interrelationships guide the context in which care should be provided. The primary direction should be the integration of evidenced-based decision-making through shared professional collaborations. If these professions continue practicing in silos, the primary competency of providing patient-centered care will not be fully implemented, and the best patient outcomes will not be achieved. The committee agreed with the plan based on interprofessional education in the policy committee meetings.

Strategy: Systematic Step-by-Step Educational Content

The next committee session began with the use of the seven steps of the EBP process (Melnyk, Fineout-Overholt, Stillwell, & Williamson, 2010) and the EBP competencies as tools to guide the step-by-step development of the committee's EBP knowledge and skills (for more information about the seven-step EBP process, see Chapter 1):

- The consultant began by leading a discussion on the importance of an ongoing curiosity about the best evidence to guide clinical decision-making (Step #0 of the EBP process). She asked the committee to provide examples of patient care procedures or policies that stimulated questions in their practice. A culture of EBP allows opportunity to question why patient care procedures are practiced in certain ways. Comfort in asking questions is present in a supportive culture (Melnyk et al., 2010). The consultant asked them to bring a clinical question related to practice with them for the next session.

- The committee reviewed the systematic way to ask a clinical question and why PICOT is important (Step #1 of the EBP process). The consultant had the committee members practice developing their own clinical questions in PICOT format for all to see. They critiqued each other's questions. She and the chair worked with members individually during the meeting and were available after the meeting. Additionally, the consultant was available via email or telephone between the meetings for individual consultation.

- The NCH Manager of Library Services provided a program on searching databases for research, best practices, and standards of practice upon which clinical decisions may be made (Step #2 of the EBP process). She demonstrated how to select keywords from the PICOT question and how to limit the search to specific practices. The use of the electronic library and searching available resources were reviewed in depth. The committee provided examples of topics, and she provided brief searches as examples. Levels of evidence and determining the validity of the information was presented. She also discussed the evidence-based library services that are available through the hospital and its affiliation with The Ohio State University Library. Members commented that they did not know about the comprehensive library services available to them.

- Multiple sessions were dedicated to critically appraising the evidence (Step #3 of the EBP process) by selecting an appropriate template provided by the consultant. The committee was asked to bring an article to use for critical appraisal practice. The consultant provided examples of how to determine the highest quality of evidence available and reviewed sample articles for the type of research. Reviewing the difference between evaluation/summary and synthesis required two meetings. Walking the committee through creating synthesis tables from the selected articles and selecting the articles that pertained to the clinical question took considerable time. Participants identified specific policies that were in need of practice changes, developed PICOT questions, interacted with an evidence-based practice librarian who used keywords from PICOT questions as samples for literature searches, critically appraised the evidence, and developed synthesis tables.

- The committee discussed the importance of seeking evidence that pertained to pediatric practice and incorporating family and patient preferences into clinical practice decisions (Step #4 of the EBP process).

- Incorporating EBP into quality improvement (QI) processes was discussed (Step #5 of the EBP process). The organization has a large structure to support QI activities. The committee reported that taking the time to incorporate EBP into QI processes to change practice could improve trial-and-error approaches.

- The chair and consultant presented the project at the Sigma Theta Tau International Research Congress in 2015 (Step #6 of the EBP process).

Operationalizing the EBP Education Project

To facilitate the educational program, steps were taken to adapt current policy committee schedules and communications:

- EBP education time was scheduled during the meetings when the group was together. The members felt they could not dedicate time outside the meetings due to their schedules and could not take time for an external immersion class as a group or individually.

- The administrative activities navigated by the chair included reorganizing the committee meeting schedules/agendas to incorporate the education sessions without adding a substantial amount of time.

- The chair and consultant agreed to communicate via telephone and email to plan the details. Adapting the program to the pace of the committee was critical.

- The consultant's assistant coordinated the appointments for the communications and meetings.

- Most meetings included 1 hour of time spent in sessions on the steps of EBP and discussions on the practical application of the steps.

- Innovative ways to carve out time for EBP competency education evolved. Online review/voting of less-complicated policies saved time; routine reviews that recommend no or few changes in policy or practice also were appropriate for online review.

- Each education session began with a brief review of previous steps and discussions.

- When the committee agenda was heavy or when the consultant was not available, the entire meeting was devoted to committee business. Flexibility in operationalizing the plan was important.

CHALLENGES TO USING THE EVIDENCE-BASED PRACTICE COMPETENCIES WITH POLICY AND PROCEDURE COMMITTEES

Committees always have several challenges facing them. In the case of implementing EBP competencies, these challenges included how to find time to add topics to agendas, keep all members interested and participating, and agree on policy changes.

Integrating EBP Education Sessions Into Committee Business Meetings

Timely processing of practice changes requires a tight schedule for review of policies. The committee oversees 286 policies, not including attachments, and reviewing each one requires a minimum of every 3 years; however, many policy reviews occur much more often as practice or regulations change. Compressing the business meeting to 1 hour to make room for EBP education sessions required meeting efficiency from the chair and committee.

When the demand for review of many policies dominated the agenda, the session was postponed until the next month. When the agenda was less demanding, additional time was arranged with the consultant. Flexibility and a positive outlook on the value of juggling the business meeting with the EBP sessions were needed to continue through the process. The sessions were intentionally scheduled over many months, and the committee agreed that the benefit of a continual education process over time would help enculturate the EBP processes into the work of the committee.

Committee Member Variation of Interest in the EBP Project

Active committee member participation varied. Interprofessional members had busy schedules, and a few chose not to participate in the survey initially. Occasionally, some members missed the education sessions when their jobs required them to be in multiple meetings or to cover duties in a clinical area. Some were very attentive and asked questions and completed homework and PICOT questions in advance of the meeting. A few expressed concerns whether they should remain on the committee or whether they had the time to spend on EBP. The chair received comments related to the time needed to follow the EBP steps.

The time spent in the committee meetings was supported by the organization; however, time spent outside committee meetings had to be worked into the usual day-to-day work schedule of the committee member. Members reported lack of time to search for articles that was complicated by the need for evidence specifically related to pediatric practice concerns. Yoder, Kirkley, Kirksey, StalBaum, and Sellers (2014) found that many nurses recognize the importance of applying evidence, but indicated they needed assistance in locating evidence. This trend was seen at this hospital when some committee members reported that they expected unit-based educators or advanced practice registered nurses (APRNs) to locate, analyze, and synthesize the evidence for them. Several members of the committee expressed doubt whether they would be able to develop the skills themselves. Another challenge was that when clinical expert staff were expected to perform the steps needed in EBP along with their usual clinical responsibilities, release time was not budgeted in many areas.

The critical appraisal step was the greatest challenge. Time to learn how to critically appraise articles and time to integrate the information into pediatric practice were reported as major barriers to following the EBP steps. Leading discussions with other stakeholders also was challenging. Simply sending emails to peers was not enough effort to elicit involvement of clinical experts outside the committee.

Changes in Committee Membership

A few members resigned from the committee and project due to changing positions, leaving the organization, or being replaced with another clinical representative from their area. Incoming new members did not have a formal process for orientation and had to jump in and catch up with the program. There was an ongoing need for the chair to explain the project to new members or to those with poor attendance.

Outcomes of Committee Processes

Committee processes began to change. The Patient/Family Policy Committee members began to refine their EBP skills and modeled the use of EBP to the clinical experts on their policy teams. Examples of outcomes include:

- The charter for the committee was reviewed at the beginning of the project. During a routine review, it had been recently updated to include expectations of evidence-based practice, but the actualization of the practice had not been consistently implemented. The review at the beginning of the project was helpful to reinforce the need for enculturation through education. As the project progressed, the chair began to feel they were speaking the language of evidence-based practice.

- Committee process checklists recently developed but not consistently implemented began to be incorporated into the steps of policy review as guides to the expected incorporation of evidence. The committee members began to distribute the checklist with a cover letter to anyone expressing interest in a new policy or policy change.

- One point of clarification was to review and agree on the purpose of the committee Policy XI-00:10 Policy, Procedure, Protocol, and Guidelines Standards (Nationwide Children's Hospital, 2014), a policy that guides expectations of staff related to basic safe patient care. It includes rules on identification of patients, comfort measures, patient/family education, and family-centered care. The policy defines the purpose of the Patient/Family Care Policy Committee Manual. The EBP statement from the policy follows:

   The policy, procedure, protocols and guidelines content in the Patient/ family Care Policy Committee Manual is designed to provide specific information that the caregiver needs to practice safe and efficient Family Centered care within Nationwide Children's Hospital. Policies, procedures, protocols and guidelines will be supported by evidence such as research, best practices, regulatory criteria and professional literature.

DEVELOPMENT OF A UNIT-BASED EBP POLICY: A PERSONAL NARRATIVE

A unit-based education specialist that had been a member of the hospital's Patient/Family Care Policy Committee for more than 8 years and was participating in the EBP Competency Study as well as educational sessions was assigned a policy update and challenged to use the step-by-step process. The educator does not specifically remember learning about evidence-based practice from the late 1980s while working on a bachelor's degree in nursing; however, research was important in her nursing curriculum at that time. While in graduate school in the late 1990s, she remembers that research was even more important in her education. There was a requirement to complete a research project and write a thesis. Reflecting back, she thought she had worked on "evidence-based practice."

When the hospital Patient/Family Care Policy Committee discussed providing evidence to guide the policies and procedures that were being reviewed, revised, and developed, she thought she knew what that entailed. She would find several articles that supported the information in the policy and felt good that she could do what was required. Little did she know that she was merely providing publications. She realized she needed to learn the difference between research, quality improvement, and evidence-based practice, and how each of these plays a role in the development of hospital policies and procedures.

Having been a nurse at Nationwide Children's Hospital for 25 years, 16 of which were in unit-based education, she became the education specialist on a 24-bed pediatric surgery unit where she is responsible for all aspects of staff education. The unit provides specialty care for patients with short bowel syndrome, post-operative bariatric patients, post-operative renal transplant donors, and a variety of general post-operative surgical patients.

In alignment with the NCH strategic plan, a new colorectal and pelvic reconstruction surgeon had been recruited to expand care into a complex colorectal patient population. Although the staff were experienced in post-operative surgery care, this new physician and complex patient population brought many practice changes and staff education challenges.

One of the first assignments for this educator after the beginning of the EBP policy committee education project was to oversee the review of the hospital policy on the enema procedure. She thought this would be a simple policy to begin EBP policy review. The enema procedure was new, and she thought that the "evidence" would be easy to find and explain. She used the committee template for reviewing the policy that included a checklist for assuring hospital departments from a variety of settings review the policy for accuracy and recommend needed revisions that apply to their respective areas. The educator was reminded that the new colorectal clinic would be using the policy as its new method for administering an enema, including using a balloon catheter. She discovered that procedures within the hospital system differed, and nonstandardization was in conflict with the hospital patient safety philosophy. This provided a great opportunity to demonstrate how evidence was necessary to guide clinical practice and ensure all areas of the hospital are practicing using a standardized policy and procedure.

The colorectal program's APRN partnered with the educator to provide "evidence" to support the new enema procedure using the balloon catheter. The proposed changes to the enema procedure along with the evidence were presented to the various affected services and stakeholders from multiple areas. They agreed the changes where appropriate. The changes to the policy were made and approved at the policy committee meeting.

The educator worked with the hospital's Professional Development Department to provide the education about the policy changes to the staff on all units. Several nursing leaders did not feel comfortable with the updated practices in the policy and did not want to implement the practice changes. The changes had been based on the best evidence available, including physician clinical expertise and preferences, but high-level, randomized controlled trials were not available. It was now even clearer that the seven-step process of EBP was critical. However, more discussion about the evidence was needed before some of the stakeholders could accept the changes.

The following is a summary of how the team utilized the steps of EBP (Melnyk & Fineout-Overholt, 2011) and how they worked with the enema policy revisions:

- The need for EBP to guide hospital policy was cultivated within the inter-professional policy committee. As the hospital continues to grow and strive for excellence in patient care, it is imperative to champion EBP, and also that staff are adequately educated (Step #0 of the EBP process).

- The PICOT question evolved throughout the EBP process (Step #1). It was necessary to revise the PICOT several times to help search for evidence. There was no specific T (time) for this question.

  - *Initial PICO:* In pediatric patients receiving an enema (P), how does the use of a balloon catheter (I) compared to not using a balloon catheter (C) affect enema results (O)?

  - *Final PICO:* In pediatric patients receiving an enema (P), how does the use of a balloon-type catheter (I) compared to using a traditional rectal tube (C) affect fecal continence (O)?

- It was difficult to find evidence about the best way to provide the enema procedure, especially in the pediatric population (Step #2). Utilizing the expertise of the trained librarians, several articles were found to guide this project. Of the multiple articles reviewed, seven were selected as keeper articles. Two of the studies found were greater than 5 years old, two were 5 years old, five were conducted in countries outside the United States, and five looked into the care of children.

- Learning the skill of critical appraisal is an ongoing process (Step #3). It takes significant time while learning but does improve with practice. The limited evidence on this topic and lower-level evidence made this important step in EBP even more challenging.

- As discussed in Melnyk and Fineout-Overholt (2011), EBP integrates the best evidence from high-level studies with a clinician's expertise and a patient's preferences and values (Step #4). The evidence provided some valuable information that informed the practice change, and when combined with the clinical expertise of the colorectal surgeon and his experience with using the enema procedure in his practice and the verbalized success of more than hundreds of patients and their families (Bischoff, Levit, & Pena, 2009), the evidence-based change was implemented.

- The "so-what" outcomes of the policy change (Step #5) included:

  - An improvement in a patient's quality of life. Patients can stay cleaner for a longer period of time, which improves psychosocial interactions and confidence.

  - An increase in patient/family satisfaction with improved enema results.

  - A decrease in a patient's healthcare costs with an improvement in a patient's overall bowel health.

  - A decrease in a patient's need for hospitalization and decreasing lost days of school or work.

  - Gathering the extensive data for this step is still in progress.

- Poster presentations, podium presentations, and publications regarding this journey are in process (Step #6). An email sent by the Professional Development Specialist who disseminates policy changes to leadership and staff announced the policy changes through an SBAR.

Barriers found in the literature (Melnyk & Fineout-Overholt, 2015; Melnyk et al., 2012) that were experienced during the enema policy project included:

- Timelines

- Stakeholders with conflicting ideas

- Knowledge of EBP/EBP competencies

- Multiple PICOT questions within one policy/procedure

- Evidence not available, or minimal, for specific pediatric topics

- Access to EBP mentors/resources at the hospital

Changes in Attitudes

Near the end of the critical appraisal step, a practice activity stimulated committee reflection on the experience. The question was, "What are your thoughts about the EBP Interprofessional Education Project?" Answers reported by committee member roles are included in Table 12.2.

TABLE 12.2 FEEDBACK ON THE EBP INTERPROFESSIONAL EDUCATION PROJECT BY COMMITTEE MEMBERS

Role	Comment
Nurse Epidemiologist	*Forces you to look at evidence and not just what the group thinks; having the project last over a longer period of time reinforces EBP*
Nurse Clinical VP	*Struggle to get others to look at evidence; must look at literature ahead of time before discussing policy changes; benefit is bringing clinical experts along on their practice; leads to more involvement of frontline staff; I have a standard to involve stakeholders in the evidence and have subgroups of expert stakeholders looking at the evidence*
Social Work Director	*More exposure to early adopters when reviewing as a group; having the project occur over time helps develop a routine*
Respiratory Therapy Manager	*EBP valuable but takes a lot of time; have to believe it is important; time is the barrier; PICOT helps me focus on the problem and guide the literature search but there are multiple PICOT questions in each clinical practice policy update*
Pharmacy Manager	*This EBP project is eye-opening; I will be using more librarian time (now that I know their expertise); still struggle with my own literature search skills; I need more search strategies (like the librarians); everyday practice should marry innovation and EBP*
Education Nurse Specialist	*Policies need to be applicable to practice and this process helps; stressful due to level of detail needed; I am thinking differently about needing evidence for practice; trying to find time to mentor others; some others find superficial evidence without critically appraising the study*

Moving Ahead

As the committee neared the end of the project, a discussion that was held on how to move forward and further enculturate the steps of EBP into committee operations resulted in these newly developed beliefs about the committee and EBP. In the past, EBP had been a lower priority in the processing of policy/procedure review, and now EBP is a higher priority. Lessons learned through the project implementation include:

- **Structural**

  - A role description for members is needed that includes EBP.

  - Committee members' EBP responsibilities require an allocation of time to coordinate the EBP steps with their team and stakeholders.

  - Clarifying importance of attendance helps ensure interprofessional involvement.

  - Setting priorities on time and effort to focus on evidence-based procedures is beneficial.

  - Many policies are regulatory rules or internal rules used to clarify roles, responsibilities, and structure of patient care and may not need to be evidence-based.

  - Dedicated time is needed to work on EBP projects.

- **Process**

  - Use the seven EBP steps to guide the policy revision process.

  - Take the time needed to assure review and revisions are evidence-based.

  - Keeping committee members onboard.

  - Members will have to be more diligent to include stakeholders.

  - Members will have to be more diligent to follow the steps of EBP.

  - Monitor the internal politics of engaging key stakeholders.

  - Manage change process.

- Set priorities on time and effort to focus on evidence-based procedures.

- Educate stakeholders and peers as you go.

- **EBP Enculturation**

  - As an organization that values quality and safety in patient care, the committee should make enculturating the processes and modeling the EBP practices with peers and stakeholders a priority.

  - Exposure to the details of the EBP process will lead to evidence-based policies/procedures and the improvement of quality and safety in patient care.

  - Realize that the old way of policy/procedure management and review was trial and error.

  - Recognition of the value of EBP.

  - Focus on the "so-what" outcomes in discussions with stakeholders.

SUMMARY

Early steps that facilitated the project included having a leader with a vision for EBP, identifying internal and external resources, nurturing academic partner relationships, and developing time- and cost-efficient methods to incorporate EBP education and mentoring. Improving the EBP knowledge and skills of the policy and procedure committee members by integrating EBP education into committee meetings not only instilled more EBP into the patient care policies, but also increased the professional interactions among the interprofessional members. The systematic step-by-step approach over time to improve the integration of evidence into patient care policies was cost-effective and required no additional committee meetings. Committee engagement in the planning and evaluation of the project was key to buy-in of the participants. The hospital underpinnings of a high-performing organization with a dedication to excellence in safe patient care, along with a Magnet®-influenced practice environment, supported the accomplishment of the project.

REFERENCES

American Nurses Credentialing Center. (2013). *2014 Magnet® application manual.* Silver Spring, MD: American Nurses Association.

Bischoff, A., Levitt, M. A., & Pena, A. (2009). Bowel management for the treatment of pediatric fecal incontinence. *Pediatric Surgery International, 25*(12), 1027–1042.

Institute of Medicine (IOM). (2003). *Health professions education: A bridge to quality.* Washington, DC: National Academies Press.

Institute of Medicine (U.S.) Roundtable on Evidence-Based Medicine. (2009). *Leadership commitments to improve value in healthcare: Finding common ground: Workshop summary.* Washington, DC: National Academies Press. Retrieved from http://www.ncbi.nlm.nih.gov/books/NBK52847/

Interprofessional Education Collaborative Expert Panel. (2011). *Core competencies for interprofessional collaborative practice: Report of an expert panel.* Washington, DC: Interprofessional Education Collaborative.

Melnyk, B. M., & Fineout-Overholt, E. (2011). *Evidence-based practice in nursing & healthcare: A guide to best practice* (2nd ed.). Philadelphia, PA: Wolters Kluwer/Lippincott Williams & Wilkins.

Melnyk, B. M., & Fineout-Overholt, E. (2015). *Evidence-based practice in nursing & healthcare: A guide to best practice* (3rd ed.). Philadelphia, PA: Wolters Kluwer.

Melnyk, B. M., Fineout-Overholt, E., Gallagher-Ford, L., & Kaplan, L. (2012). The state of evidence-based practice in US nurses: Critical implications for nurse leaders and educators. *Journal of Nursing Administration, 42*(9), 410–417.

Melnyk, B. M., Fineout-Overholt, E., Stillwell, S. B., & Williamson, K. M. (2010). The seven steps of evidence-based practice. *American Journal of Nursing, 110*(1), 51–53.

Melnyk, B. M., & Gallagher-Ford, L. (2014). Evidence-based practice as mission critical for healthcare quality and safety: A disconnect for many nurse executives. *Worldviews on Evidence-Based Nursing, 11,* 145–146.

Melnyk, B. M., Gallagher-Ford, L., Long, L., & Fineout-Overholt, E. (2014). The establishment of evidence-based practice competencies for practicing nurses and advanced practice nurses in real-world clinical settings: Proficiencies to improve healthcare quality, reliability, patient outcomes, and costs. *Worldviews on Evidence-Based Nursing, 11*(1), 5–15.

Nationwide Children's Hospital. (2014). Policy XI-00:10 Policy, Procedure, Protocol and Guidelines Standards.

Robert Wood Johnson Foundation. (September 2011). Health policy snapshot: Workforce. Retrieved from http://www.rwjf.org/content/dam/farm/reports/issue_briefs/2011/rwjf72058

Yoder, L. H., Kirkley, D., McFall, D. C., Kirksey, K. M., StalBaum, A. L., & Sellers, D. (2014). Staff nurses' use of research to facilitate evidence-based practice. *American Journal of Nursing, 114*(9), 26–38.

CHAPTER 13

TEACHING THE EVIDENCE-BASED PRACTICE COMPETENCIES IN CLINICAL AND ACADEMIC SETTINGS

Ellen Fineout-Overholt, PhD, RN, FNAP, FAAN;
Tracy L. Brewer, DNP, RNC-OB, CLC;
Lisa English Long, MSN, RN, CNS; and
Tina L. Magers, PhD, RN-BC

KEY CONTENT IN THIS CHAPTER

- Essential elements for teaching evidence-based practice (EBP) competencies

- Crosswalk of EBP competencies with regulatory, credentialing, and accrediting requirements in academic and clinical settings

- Strategies for teaching EBP competencies

- Strategies for learning about evaluating EBP competencies

> Excellence must be achieved through the eyes of those who judge us; once achieved it can only be maintained with constant innovation.
>
> –Tom Collins

Evidence-based practice (EBP), well established as the foundation for best practice and nursing education, is expected for the 21st century nurse (American Association of Colleges of Nursing [AACN], 2006, 2008, 2011; American Nurses Credentialing Center, 2014; Centers for Medicare & Medicaid Services, 2014; Fineout-Overholt, Stillwell, Williamson, Cox, & Robbins, 2015; Greiner & Knebel, 2003; Institute of Medicine [IOM], 1999, 2001, 2002, 2010; Joint Commission, 2013; National League for Nursing [NLN], 2012). Establishing curricula that address the required competencies in patient-centered care, interprofessional practice, EBP, quality improvement (QI), and informatics requires thoughtful reflection about its foundations, content delivery methods, and evaluation strategies (Fineout-Overholt, 2013; Fineout-Overholt & Johnston, 2005, 2007).

The EBP competencies help address these important areas. Particular attention to the language of the EBP paradigm and process as well as evidence-based decision-making (EBDM) offers learners in any setting the opportunity to be equipped to meet the expectations of today's healthcare organizations. Learners come prepared to focus on providing best care versus academic investment in a traditional focus on the conduct of research that is not carried over into their careers as nurses (Ciliska, 2005; Fineout-Overholt, 2015). The EBP competencies provide rich guidance on what curricula must include to help nurse graduates across levels (e.g., BSN, MSN, and doctoral education) to successfully engage their roles as evidence-based clinicians, leaders, and scientists.

The field of education is still evolving as to how to best teach EBP. Melnyk, Fineout-Overholt, and colleagues demonstrated that in academia, while faculty believed they were teaching EBP, often their strategies were too simplistic to establish proficiency in the EBP process or paradigm (Melnyk, Fineout-Overholt, Feinstein, Sadler, & Green-Hernandez, 2008). Coomarasamy and Khan (2004) and Moch and colleagues (2010) spoke to how often academic organizations focus on the evaluation of student work completed within academic programming yet fail to evaluate the sustainable impact of student learning beyond the classroom. Practicing nurses have reported gaps in knowledge and skills regarding how to translate evidence into practice and, thereby, enhance healthcare outcomes (Melnyk, Fineout-Overholt, Gallagher-Ford, & Kaplan, 2012; Melnyk, Fineout-Overholt, Giggleman, & Cruz, 2010; Wallen et al. 2010).

To facilitate "sticky learning" that lasts past academic engagement, there needs to be a systematic approach to teaching the EBP process. This begins with the EBP paradigm. Faculty must have this paradigm or teaching EBP versus research becomes challenging. Furthermore, as students engage EBP across educational and clinical roles/responsibilities, there must be a leveling of expectations of what knowledge and skills should be actualized. For example, BSN graduates should have a novice grasp of all seven steps of the EBP process, with more developed expertise in the first four steps (i.e., inquiry through critical appraisal) (AACN, 2008; NLN, 2012). An MSN graduate will have proficient expertise in all seven steps of the EBP process, and DNP clinicians will be expert across the entire EBP process (AACN, 2006, 2011, 2015). Nurse scientists graduating from PhD in nursing programs should have the most expertise with steps #0–4 (inquiry through critical appraisal) and guide the profession by producing readily translatable evidence for practice. Their work must be predicated on the systematic review of existing evidence for it to guide practice.

Herein lies the rub: In academia (and in some clinical settings), students and staff nurses are still expected to generate research versus implement EBP. Paradigm confusion can lead to language barriers and variations in outcome expectations (Fineout-Overholt, 2015). Consider two educators teaching the same course, with the same objectives: One faculty member focuses on research generation, calling it "EBP," and the other focuses on evidence translation, also calling it "EBP." Across academic and clinical settings, there needs to be a common language and outcomes defined for EBP. These EBP competencies meet this need. Furthermore, to teach the EBP competencies, EBDM must be taught across the curriculum, not in a single course. This approach facilitates educators teaching from the evidence. In an academic setting in which future healthcare providers are provided a foundation for their lifelong careers, these competencies offer an opportunity to have a common language and outcomes.

Another benefit to using an EBDM approach to teaching—incorporating these competencies—is this approach counters the idea of educators identifying as an outcome: "Here is what I want you to do." Incorporating these competencies within the academic and clinical setting requires a more learner-centered focus.

Learners must embrace this focus and move away from accepting being told what to do in their educational journeys. Teaching and learning techniques, such as team-based learning, offer learners the opportunity to grow into independent decision-makers—knowing how to put what they know into what they do in practice. Learners move past focusing on the assignment to focusing on living "what I know" and owning their knowledge.

Learners then actualize this worldview in their practices, whether their role in healthcare is staff, advanced practice, administration, or education. Furthermore, when this proactive worldview is actualized, other interprofessional colleagues in healthcare have realistic expectations that nurses will be active in EBP. The EBP competencies offer an opportunity for each of these contributors to healthcare to determine how they actualize the competencies in their role—how they contribute to best practice and its associated outcomes. In addition, the specific role of an EBP mentor is critical to the success of actualizing the EBP paradigm and process in any setting (Levin, Fineout-Overholt, Melnyk, Barnes, & Vetter, 2011). Often EBP mentors do not have their role designated; however, their impact on academic and clinical outcomes is nonetheless critical. For example, nursing professional development educators understand that for nurses to be effective decision-makers, they must be able to help nurses practice to the fullest extent of their role. Readily applying knowledge to anticipate and resolve clinical issues is evidence of assimilating into one's practice the EBP paradigm and use of current knowledge. These EBP mentors can quickly influence outcomes within a system, however small. The impact realized is that evidence speaks for itself and yields a convincing argument over and above opinion.

Both in the academic and clinical setting, the role of interprofessional practice is gaining momentum. Current clinical and academic standards speak to integration of interprofessional experiences into daily life (AACN, 2008, 2011; Greiner & Knebel, 2003). The basis for interprofessional practice is EBP. It provides a common framework for addressing clinical issues. Interprofessional stakeholders also provide a network for problem-solving through shared EBDM focused on achieving safe and effective patient, system, and provider outcomes.

MATCHING THE EBP COMPETENCIES TO EXISTING STANDARDS

To help actualize teaching of the EBP competencies across academic and healthcare settings, here are two crosswalk tables that match the EBP competencies with professional regulatory, credentialing, and accrediting organizations' standards (see Tables 13.1 and 13.2). In Table 13.1, these standards are categorized across levels of education as well as by the constructs upon which the standards are based. For academic learners, faculty have the responsibility of providing education that addresses the required levels of the EBP competencies and assists learners to consider how those competencies will transfer into their careers regardless of clinical setting.

In Table 13.2, Magnet® Forces (ANCC), which are indicators of excellence in patient care, and EBP competencies are matched together. The goal is for a student learner or a healthcare professional learner to function at the highest and safest level when providing quality patient care. This level of care is demonstrated in the exemplars at the end of the chapter.

Table 13.1 Teaching EBP Competencies in Academic Settings

Academic Guidance Organizations and Guiding Standard, Essential or Certification Construct	Degree or Certification	EBP Competencies to Meet	Related Organizational Requirements (e.g., standards, essentials)
			National League for Nursing (NLN)
Nursing Judgment	ADN	#1, 2, 11	• "Make judgments in practice, substantiated with evidence, that integrate nursing science in the provision of safe, quality care and promote the health of patients within a family and community context" p. 34
	BSN	#7, 9	• "Make judgments in practice, substantiated with evidence, that synthesize nursing science and knowledge from other disciplines in provision of safe, quality care and promote the health of patients within a family & communities" p. 34
	MSN	#14, 15	• "Make judgments in one's specialty area of practice that reflect a scholarly critique of current evidence from nursing & other disciplines & the capacity to identify gaps in knowledge and formulate research questions" p. 34
	DNP	#14, 15, 16, 17, 24	• "Systematically synthesize evidence from nursing and other disciplines & translate this knowledge to enhance nursing practice & the ability of nurses to make judgments in practice" p. 34
Spirit of Inquiry	ADN	#1, 5, 6, 8	• "Examine the evidence that underlies clinical nursing practice to challenge the status quo, question underlying assumptions, and offer new insights to improve the quality of care for patients, families, & communities" p. 36
	BSN	#1, 2, 3, 5, 6, 8	• "Act as an evolving scholar who contributes to the development of the science of nursing practice by identifying questions of need of study, critiquing published research, & using available evidence as a foundation to propose creative, innovative, or evidence-based solutions to clinical practice problems" p. 36
	Masters	#14, 15, 16, 19, 21	• "Contribute to the science of nursing in one's specialty area of practice by analyzing underlying disparities in knowledge or evidence; formulating research questions; & systematically evaluating the impact on quality when evidence-based solutions to nursing problems are implemented" p. 36

Academic Guidance Organizations and Guiding Standard, Essential or Certification Construct	Degree or Certification	EBP Competencies to Meet	Related Organizational Requirements (e.g., standards, essentials)
	DNP	#12	• "Disseminate practice-based knowledge by engaging in practice with an open mind; systematically studying the practice of other nurses; & reviewing extant research to formulate evidence-based proposals enhancing nursing practice, education, or the delivery of nursing services" p. 36
American Association of Colleges of Nursing (AACN)			
Essential III: Scholarship for Evidence-Based Practice	BSN	#1–13	• Explain the interrelationships among theory, practice, and research • Demonstrate an understanding of the basic elements of the research process and models for applying evidence to clinical practice • Advocate for the protection of human subjects in the conduct of research • Evaluate the credibility of sources of information, including but not limited to databases and Internet resources • Participate in the process of retrieval, appraisal, and synthesis of evidence in collaboration with other members of the healthcare team to improve patient outcomes • Integrate evidence, clinical judgment, interprofessional perspectives, and patient preferences in planning, implementing, and evaluating outcomes of care • Collaborate in the collection, documentation, and dissemination of evidence • Acquire an understanding of the process for how nursing and related healthcare quality and safety measures are developed, validated, and endorsed • Describe mechanisms to resolve identified practice discrepancies between identified standards and practice that may adversely impact patient outcomes
Essential IV: Translating and Integrating Scholarship into Practice	Masters	#1–24	• Integrate theory, evidence, clinical judgment, research, and interprofessional perspectives using translational processes to improve practice and associated health outcomes for patient aggregates • Advocate for the ethical conduct of research and translational scholarship (with particular attention to the protection of the patient as a research participant) • Articulate to a variety of audiences the evidence base for practice decisions,

continues

Table 13.1 Teaching EBP Competencies in Academic Settings (continued)

Academic Guidance Organizations and Guiding Standard, Essential or Certification Construct	Degree or Certification	EBP Competencies to Meet	Related Organizational Requirements (e.g., standards, essentials)
			including the credibility of sources of information and the relevance to the practice problem confronted • Participate, leading when appropriate, in collaborative teams to improve care outcomes and support policy changes through knowledge generation, knowledge dissemination, and planning and evaluating knowledge implementation • Apply practice guidelines to improve practice and the care environment • Perform rigorous critique of evidence derived from databases to generate meaningful evidence for nursing practice
Essential III: Clinical Scholarship and Analytical Methods for Evidence-Based Practice	DNP	#1–24	• Use analytic methods to critically appraise existing literature and other evidence to determine and implement the best evidence for practice • Design and implement processes to evaluate outcomes of practice, practice patterns, and systems of care within a practice setting, healthcare organization, or community against national benchmarks to determine variances in practice outcomes and population trends • Design, direct, and evaluate quality improvement methodologies to promote safe, timely, effective, efficient, equitable, and patient-centered care • Apply relevant findings to develop practice guidelines and improve practice and the practice environment • Use information technology and research methods appropriately • Function as a practice specialist/consultant in collaborative knowledge-generating research • Disseminate findings from evidence-based practice and research to improve healthcare outcomes

Academic Guidance Organizations and Guiding Standard, Essential or Certification Construct	Degree or Certification	EBP Competencies to Meet	Related Organizational Requirements (e.g., standards, essentials)
AACN Competencies and Curricular Expectations for Clinical Nurse Leader			
Essential 4: Translating and Integrating Scholarship into Practice	Clinical Nurse Leader	#1–24	• Facilitate practice change based on best available evidence that results in quality, safety & fiscally responsible outcomes • Ensure the inclusion of an ethical decision-making framework for quality improvement • Implement strategies for encouraging a culture of inquiry within the healthcare delivery team • Facilitate the process of retrieval, appraisal, & synthesis of evidence in collaboration with healthcare team members, including patients, to improve care outcomes • Communicate to the interprofessional healthcare team, patients, & caregivers current quality & safety guidelines & nurse sensitive indicators, including the endorsement & validation processes • Apply improvement science theory & methods in performance measurement & quality improvement process • Lead change initiatives to decrease or eliminate discrepancies between actual practices and identified standards of care • Disseminate changes in practice & improvements in care outcomes to internal & external audiences • Design care based on outcome analysis & evidence to promote safe, timely, effective, efficient, equitable & patient-centered care
National Organization of Nurse Practitioner Faculties (NONPF)			
Practice Inquiry	Nurse Practitioner	#1–24	• Provide leadership in the translation of new knowledge into practice • Generate knowledge from clinical practice to improve practice and patient outcomes • Apply clinical investigative skills to improve health outcomes • Lead practice inquiry, individually or in partnership with others • Disseminate evidence from inquiry to diverse audiences using multiple modalities • Analyze clinical guidelines for individualized application into practice

continues

Table 13.1 Teaching EBP Competencies in Academic Settings (continued)

Academic Guidance Organizations and Guiding Standard, Essential or Certification Construct	Degree or Certification	EBP Competencies to Meet	Related Organizational Requirements (e.g., standards, essentials)
National Association of Clinical Nurse Specialists (NACNS)			

Research Competency: Interpretation, Translation & Use of Evidence	CNS	#1–24	• Analyze research findings & other evidence for their potential application to clinical practice
			• Integrate evidence into the health, illness, & wellness management of patients, families, communities, and groups
			• Apply principles of EBP & quality improvement to all patient care
			• Assess barriers & facilitators to adoption of EBP
			• Design programs for effective implementation of research findings & other evidence in clinical practice
			• Cultivate a climate of clinical inquiry across spheres of influence:
			  ○ Evaluates the need for improvement or redesign of care delivery processes to improve safety, efficiency, reliability, and quality
			  ○ Disseminates expert knowledge

Nursing Education			
Nurse Educator Competencies: Knowledge, Skills & Attitudes	Nurse Educator	#1–24	• Ground teaching strategies in educational theory and evidence-based teaching practices • Use information technologies skillfully to support the teaching-learning process • Model critical and reflective thinking • Create opportunities for learners to develop their critical thinking and clinical reasoning skills • Maintain the professional practice knowledge base needed to help learners prepare for contemporary nursing practice

Academic Guidance Organizations and Guiding Standard, Essential or Certification Construct	Degree or Certification	EBP Competencies to Meet	Related Organizational Requirements (e.g., standards, essentials)
American Organization of Nurse Executives (AONE)			
Knowledge of the Healthcare Environment: EBP/Outcome Measurement Communication & Relationship Building: Shared Decision Making	Nurse Executive	#1–24	• Interpret information from research • Utilize research findings for the establishment of standards, practices, & patient care models in the organization • Disseminate research findings to patient care team members • Participate in studies that provide outcome measurements • Allocate nursing resources based on measurement of patient acuity/care needed • Engage staff and others in decision-making • Promote decisions that are patient-centered • Provide an environment conducive to opinion-sharing
Quality and Safety Education for Nurses (QSEN)			
Pre-licensure	Knowledge	#1, 4, 5, 6, 7	• Demonstrate knowledge of basic scientific methods and processes • Describe EBP to include the components of research evidence, clinical expertise and patient/family values • Differentiate clinical opinion from research and evidence summaries • Describe reliable sources for locating evidence reports and clinical practice guidelines • Explain the role of evidence in determining best clinical practice • Describe how the strength and relevance of available evidence influences the choice of interventions in provision of patient-centered care • Discriminate between valid and invalid reasons for modifying evidence-based clinical practice based on clinical expertise or patient/family preferences
	Skills	#1–10	• Participate effectively in appropriate data collection and other research activities • Adhere to Institutional Review Board (IRB) guidelines

continues

Table 13.1 Teaching EBP Competencies in Academic Settings (continued)

Academic Guidance Organizations and Guiding Standard, Essential or Certification Construct	Degree or Certification	EBP Competencies to Meet	Related Organizational Requirements (e.g., standards, essentials)
Pre-licensure	Skills	#1–10	• Base individualized care plan on patient values, clinical expertise and evidence • Read original research and evidence reports related to area of practice • Locate evidence reports related to clinical practice topics and guidelines • Participate in structuring the work environment to facilitate integration of new evidence into standards of practice • Question rationale for routine approaches to care that result in less-than-desired outcomes or adverse events • Consult with clinical experts before deciding to deviate from evidence-based protocols
Graduate	Knowledge	#1–24	• Demonstrate knowledge of health research methods and processes • Describe evidence-based practice to include the components of research evidence, clinical expertise and patient/family values • Identify efficient and effective search strategies to locate reliable sources of evidence • Identify principles that comprise the critical appraisal of research evidence • Summarize current evidence regarding major diagnostic and treatment actions within the practice specialty • Determine evidence gaps within the practice specialty • Analyze how the strength of available evidence influences the provision of care (assessment, diagnosis, treatment and evaluation) • Evaluate organizational cultures and structures that promote evidence-based practice

Academic Guidance Organizations and Guiding Standard, Essential or Certification Construct	Degree or Certification	EBP Competencies to Meet	Related Organizational Requirements (e.g., standards, essentials)
Graduate	Skills		• Use health research methods and processes, alone or in partnership with scientists, to generate new knowledge for practice • Adhere to Institutional Review Board guidelines • Role-model clinical decision-making based on evidence, clinical expertise and patient/family preferences and values • Employ efficient and effective search strategies to answer focused clinical questions • Critically appraise original research and evidence summaries related to area of practice • Exhibit contemporary knowledge of best evidence related to practice specialty • Promote research agenda for evidence that is needed in practice specialty • Initiate changes in approaches to care when new evidence warrants evaluation of other options for improving outcomes or decreasing adverse events • Develop guidelines for clinical decision-making regarding departure from established protocols/standards of care • Participate in designing systems that support evidence-based practice

NLN (2012), AACN (2008, 2011, 2006, 2013), NONPF (2012), NACNS (2008), Halstead (2007), AONE (2015), QSEN (2007, 2009)

Table 13.2 Teaching EBP Competencies in Clinical Settings

Magnet® Recognition Components*	EBP Competencies		Related Magnet® Recognition Components
Transformational Leadership (TL)	#2:	Describes clinical problems using internal evidence	TL7: Nurse leaders, with clinical nurse input, use trended data to acquire necessary resources to support the care delivery system(s).
	#8:	Collects practice data systematically as internal evidence for clinical decision making in the care of individuals, groups, and populations	
Structural Empowerment (SE)	#16:	Integrates a body of external evidence from nursing and related fields with internal evidence in making decisions about patient care	SE1EO: Clinical nurses are involved in interprofessional decision-making groups at the organizational level.
	#20:	Formulates EBP policies and procedures	
	#24:	Communicates best evidence to individuals, groups, colleagues, and policy makers	
	#24:	Communicates best evidence to individuals, groups, colleagues, and policy makers	SE9: The organization supports nurses' participation in community healthcare outreach.
Exemplary Professional Practice (EP)	#10:	Implements practice changes based on evidence and clinical expertise and patient preferences to improve care processes and patient outcomes	EP4: Nurses create partnerships with patients and families to establish goals and plans for the delivery of patient-centered care.
	#9:	Integrates evidence gathered from external and internal sources in order to plan evidence-based practice changes	EP5: Nurses are involved in interprofessional collaborative practice within the care delivery system to ensure care coordination and continuity of care.
	#16:	Integrates a body of external evidence from nursing and related fields with internal evidence in making decisions about patient care	EP8EO: Nurses use internal and external experts to improve the clinical practice setting.

Magnet® Recognition Components*	EBP Competencies	Related Magnet® Recognition Components
	#4: Searches for external evidence to answer focused clinical questions	EP6: Nurses incorporate regulatory and specialty standards/guidelines into the development and implementation of the care delivery system.
	#9: Integrates evidence gathered from external and internal sources in order to plan evidence-based practice changes	
	#14: Systematically conducts an exhaustive search for external evidence to answer clinical questions	
	#15: Critically appraises relevant pre-appraised evidence and primary studies, including evaluation and synthesis	
	#5: Participates in critical appraisal of pre-appraised evidence	EP7EO: Nurses systematically evaluate professional organizations' standards of practice, incorporating them into the organization's professional practice model and care delivery system.
	#9: Integrates evidence gathered from external and internal sources in order to plan evidence-based practice changes	EP8EO: Nurses use internal and external experts to improve the clinical practice setting.
	#15: Critically appraises relevant pre-appraised evidence and primary studies, including evaluation and synthesis	
	#9: Integrates evidence gathered from external and internal sources in order to plan evidence-based practice changes	EP8EO: Nurses use internal and external experts to improve the clinical practice setting.
	#16: Integrates a body of external evidence from nursing and related fields with internal evidence in making decisions about patient care	
	#17: Leads transdisciplinary team in applying synthesized evidence to initiate clinical decisions and practice changes to improve the health of individuals, groups, and populations	EP12: Nurses assume leadership roles in collaborative interprofessional activities to improve the quality of care.

continues

Table 13.2 Teaching EBP Competencies in Clinical Settings (continued)

Magnet® Recognition Components*	EBP Competencies	Related Magnet® Recognition Components
	#24: Communicates best evidence to individuals, groups, colleagues, and policy makers	EP12: Nurses assume leadership roles in collaborative interprofessional activities to improve the quality of care.
	#16: Integrates a body of external evidence from nursing and related fields with internal evidence in making decisions about patient care	EP14: Resources, such as professional literature, are available to support decision making in autonomous nursing practice.
	#20: Formulates EBP policies and procedures	
	#2: Describes clinical problems using internal evidence	EP20EO: Clinical nurses are involved in the review, action planning, and evaluation of patient safety data at the unit level.
	#8: Collects practice data systematically as internal evidence for clinical decision making in the care of individuals, groups, and populations	EP20EO: Clinical nurses are involved in the review, action planning, and evaluation of patient safety data at the unit level.
		EP22EO: Unit- or clinic-level nurse-sensitive clinical indicator data outperform the mean or median of the national database used.**
New Knowledge, Innovation & Improvement (NK)	#24: Communicates best evidence to individuals, groups, colleagues, and policy makers	NK2: Nurses disseminate the organization's nursing research findings to internal and external audiences.
	#1: Questions clinical practices for the purpose of improving the quality of care	NK3: Nurses evaluate and use evidence-based findings in their practice.
	#4: Searches for external evidence to answer focused clinical questions	
	#5: Participates in critical appraisal of pre-appraised evidence	
	#6: Participates in the critical appraisal of published research studies to determine their strength and applicability to clinical practice	

Magnet® Recognition Components*	EBP Competencies	Related Magnet® Recognition Components
	#7: Participates in the evaluation and synthesis of a body of evidence gathered to determine its strength and applicability to clinical practice	
	#8: Collects practice data systematically as internal evidence for clinical decision making in the care of individuals, groups, and populations	
	#9: Integrates evidence gathered from external and internal sources in order to plan evidence-based practice changes	
	#10: Implements practice changes based on evidence and clinical expertise and patient preferences to improve care processes and patient outcomes	

*2014 Manual

**Such as falls with injury, hospital-acquired pressure ulcers stages 2 and above, central line–associated bloodstream infection, catheter-associated urinary tract infections, core measure sets

TL: transformational leadership; EP: exemplary professional practice; SE: structural empowerment; NK: new knowledge, innovation, and improvements; EO: empirical outcome

TEACHING AND EVALUATION STRATEGIES FOR INCORPORATING THE EBP COMPETENCIES

Shifting focus to educators, aligning the EBP competencies and the organizational standards can guide faculty in developing curricula, programs of study, and course assignments. Table 13.3 provides examples of teaching and evaluation strategies for teaching EBP competencies that facilitate evaluation of outcome as well as construction of course content.

A sample rubric is provided in Table 13.4 to provide one example of how discussion boards could be evaluated for evidence of EBP competencies.

Connecting the EBP competencies with regulatory, credentialing, and accrediting standards enables faculty, students, and clinicians to make the parallels that move the EBP competencies from academic or clinical "requirements" to their assimilation into the lived experience of those who will care for patients, families, communities, and populations for generations to come.

Table 13.3 Examples of Teaching and Evaluation Strategies for Selected Competencies

Competency	Activity	Outcome	Evaluation
#1: Questions clinical practices for the purpose of improving the quality of care. #2: Describes clinical problems using internal evidence.	Discussion board: • Begin initial post. State the clinical issue using either a paragraph or bullet points. • Respond to two colleagues' clinical issues.	The clinical issue is clearly described from a clinical practice perspective: "What is happening in the clinical setting that causes concern?"	Use of rubric for grading (10- or 20-point rubric)
#3: Participates in the development of clinical questions using PICOT format.	Discussion board: • Post individual PICOT questions based on clinical issue. • Respond and critique two colleagues to improve format of PICOT question.	The PICOT question is clearly stated: non-directional, "P" and "O" match, use of "how does?", "O" is measurable.	Use of rubric for grading (10- or 20-point rubric)
#4: Systematically searches for external evidence to answer focused clinical questions.	• Conduct a systematic search using PICOT question. • State databases searched. • State the final yield obtained from search.	Search strategy demonstrates a systematic approach, including keywords from PICOT question, same approach across databases.	Screen captures of systematic search in each database
#5: Participates in critical appraisal of pre-appraised evidence (such as clinical practice guidelines, evidence-based policies and procedures, and evidence syntheses). #6: Participates in the critical appraisal of published research studies to determine their strength and applicability to clinical practice.	As a group, using a known body of evidence:* • Use appropriate RCA checklists to identify keeper studies. • For keeper studies, enter study data into evaluation table. • Extract relevant data from evaluation table for synthesis tables. • Make recommendations and provide graded ratings to support recommendation.	Recommendations are relevant to clinical practice and are from the gestalt of study findings (not the researchers' conclusions).	• Have precompleted RCA checklists, evaluation table, synthesis tables, and recommendations to compare to group's. • Assess the flow from RCA checklist to recommendation: The case for the recommendation must clearly be from the evidence.
#12: Disseminates best practices supported by evidence to improve quality of care and patient outcomes.	Discussion board: • Post opportunities for disseminating EBP work in your area of practice: shared governance councils, nursing grand rounds, local, state, and national conferences.	Opportunities are identified for sharing EBP findings, information, and outcomes of change.	• Creates voiced-over poster presentation of EBP project. • Presents written plan for implementing an EBP Model with evidence-based interventions aimed at sustainable change.

*For more on RCA checklists and evaluation and synthesis tables, see Chapter 5.

Table 13.4 Sample Grading Rubric for Discussion Board: Point Value of 20

Content	Yes 4 Points	Somewhat 2 Points	Minimal 1 Point	No 0 Points	Comments
Quality, Style of Writing	Excellent grammar and syntax; accurate use of terms; no spelling errors; clearly and concisely expresses self.	Grammar, syntax and word accuracy good; some misspelled words.	Grammar, syntax and word accuracy poor; multiple misspelled words.	Does not post	
Contribution	Furthers the discussion with questions or statements that encourage others to respond. Participates with required number of postings.	Participates, but does not post in manner that encourages others to respond to posting. Participates with required number of postings.	Does not further any discussions. Less than required number of postings.	Does not post	
Professional Communication	Clearly connects posting to professional practice and discussion board theme. Writes in a tone that is consistent with professional practice and respectful to colleagues, regardless of opinions. Discussions scholarly without use of social media terms, style or slang (i.e.: LOL, C U L8er).	Some connection to professional practice/ discussion board topic. Tone needs to be more professional. Use of at least one instance of social media terms, style or slang. Respectful of differing opinions.	Mentions professional practice but no link to topic; primarily relies on informal style, tone or social media slang. Lack of respect for differing opinions.	Does not post	
Relevance	Clear reference to assignment or prior posting being discussed.	Some reference to topic; reference not within context and not understood by readers.	Posting does not clearly reflect the assignment; comments	Does not post	
			Irrelevant and off-point.		
Evidence	Course readings or data from scholarly sources cited in responses to address issue.	Inaccurately cites readings/scholarly sources in responses to address issue.		Does not post	

© Long & The Ohio State University, 2012

A REAL-WORLD EXAMPLE

TEACHING EBP COMPETENCIES #1, #2, AND #3 FOR UNDERGRADUATE STUDENTS

Dr. Jacob was assigned to teach Nursing 215, "Introduction to Evidence-based Practice." The students in this class are in the first semester of their nursing program and also are taking the "Introduction to Nursing" course (i.e., Nursing 200), which is the first course in the nursing program and is taught by Dr. Jule. Drs. Jacob and Jule discussed collaborating on an assignment for the students to achieve a learning experience that integrated the clinical experiences with the EBP course content. An additional goal provided the students the opportunity to address competencies #1, #2, and #3: (#1) questions clinical practices for the purpose of improving the quality of care; (#2) describes clinical problems using internal evidence; and (#3) participates in the formulation of clinical questions using PICOT format.

The students began their clinical experience within the first 2 weeks of the semester. In Nursing 200, an initial priority goal was to promote student inquiry related to patient experiences in the clinical setting. Week 1 of the course content focused on the history and professionalism of nursing as a discipline. Week 2 built upon the work of Florence Nightingale and her spirit of inquiry related to her experiences and inquisitive mind as she provided care to soldiers in the Crimean War. In week 3, the students began to focus on the knowledge and skills needed in providing care as they entered the clinical setting. Drs. Jule and Jacob worked together in two 3-hour consecutive days of clinical experiences during the first week when they introduced the students to healthcare organizations, care issues, and evidence-based practice. Although scheduling this time for collaboration in the setting was a challenge, each faculty identified the worth in its design in order for the students to begin thinking from a clinical inquiry perspective on day 1 of their clinical experience.

On day 1, Dr. Jule provided a tour of the organization and unit that the students would be assigned for their experiences. Throughout the tour, Dr.

continues

continued

Jacob led the students in identifying barriers and facilitators to implementation of EBP by using the OCRSIEP survey (Fineout-Overholt & Melnyk, 2006). Each student completed this survey based on a discussion with the nurse manager of the assigned unit, their observations, and information provided by faculty. The following day, students discussed their findings as well as the internal evidence that supported their findings in both pre- and post-conference with Drs. Jule and Jacob. The discussion of student findings provided faculty the opportunity to "dig deeper" into EBP and its importance in the healthcare arena, and for the students to be successful in providing the highest quality healthcare within their setting. Competency #1 was addressed in these discussions.

In weeks 3 and 4, the students completed an assignment identifying a clinical issue and why it was of interest to them and the patient and family. Identification of the issue was to be documented on an assignment sheet that asked *State the issue of concern* and *Explain why the issue is of concern*. Completing this assignment for 2 consecutive weeks allowed the students exposure to two patients, families, and reasons for hospitalization as well as application of content from lectures provided in class. When explaining the issue of concern, the students discussed why this issue was important to the patient and his/her family as well as the clinician's perspective of the issue. Dr. Jacob oversaw this aspect of the process. During these 2 weeks, competency #2 was addressed.

In weeks 5 and 6, students developed PICOT questions based on the clinical issues identified in weeks 3 and 4. Templates for developing the PICOT questions were used (Fineout-Overholt & Stillwell, 2015) by students for question formulation. The questions developed depended upon the type of issue identified by the student. PICOT questions were shared with student colleagues and Drs. Jacob and Jule in a post-conference session. Within these 2 weeks, students' work addressed competency #3.

Student completion of EBP steps and competencies that correlate to course content provides a foundation for addressing patient and family issues within an acute care setting. This foundation covers the first half of the course within one semester, allowing for next steps in the EBP process.

A REAL-WORLD EXAMPLE

TEACHING COMPETENCIES #15 AND #17 FOR ADVANCED PRACTICE NURSE GRADUATES

Professor Sanchez was assigned to teach a master's level EBP course. As a teacher in the Doctor of Nursing Practice (DNP) program, she wanted to make sure to level the content correctly when teaching EBP to MSN students. In reviewing the syllabus from her faculty colleague, she noted that the content covered in the prior term was focused on the research process. She became increasingly mindful about the focus of her teaching after reviewing Masters Essential IV (AACN, 2011), which explains that the competency of the graduate in an MSN program should relate to the translation and integration of scholarship into practice (refer to Table 13.1 for related competencies)—not conducting research.

Professor Sanchez had students in her course from different MSN concentrations, including Adult-Gerontology Acute Care Nurse Practitioner and Clinical Nurse Specialist, Pediatric Nurse Practitioner, Nurse Educator, and Nursing Administration. (Refer to Table 13.1 for specialty advance practice competencies.) To promote intradisciplinary collaboration, Professor Sanchez decided to use a teaching strategy known as *team-based learning* (TBL). She had used TBL in other courses and understood the strategy to be collaborative and interactive in which students in teams work together to solve problems that require higher-level critical thinking skills (Parmalee, Michaelson, Cook, & Hudes, 2012). Professor Sanchez was aware that for students to obtain EBP competence, they must effectively be able to work in teams. She believed that the TBL teaching strategy would be perfect for teaching an EBP course.

On the first day of class, Professor Sanchez randomly divided the students in teams that were distributed among the differing MSN concentrations. Each team had five students who quickly got to know each other and came up with a team name. Professor Sanchez explained to the students that each class would begin with an individual-readiness assurance test (iRAT)

continues

covering the content that the students were assigned to review prior to class. Students would then take the same test again as a team—the team-readiness assurance test (tRAT) (Michaelsen & Sweet, 2011). She explained that students enjoyed discussing the questions and debating the validity of the answers.

After their team came to a consensus on the correct answer, they engaged the immediate feedback assessment technique (IF-AT) by using a preprinted form that resembles a scratch-off lottery card (Epstein Educational Enterprises, n.d.), with a star showing in the scratch box if the answer is correct and a blank box for incorrect answers. After testing, Professor Sanchez explained that the students would participate in application exercises, during which the students could apply their new knowledge of the EBP process to clinical settings.

In preparing for the module on critical appraisal, Professor Sanchez decided to have the teams use the AGREE II (Brouwers et al., 2010) appraisal tool for appraising the quality of a clinical practice guideline (CPG), focusing on competency #15. Professor Sanchez recently had a DNP student who published a CPG with the National Guideline Clearinghouse (https://www. guideline.gov/) for completion of her DNP capstone project. In TBL, Professor Sanchez was aware that each team works on the same application exercise at the same time. She assigned the CPG to the student teams, and using the AGREE II tool, the students worked in teams through the critical appraisal process. They found that the process was not as easy as they anticipated after reading the chapter in their book and listening to a short online lecture. However, through collaborative discussions and varying perspectives, each team was able to appraise the quality of the guideline for use in practice. All the teams came to a consensus to recommend the guideline be used in practice, yet some students did wonder how a guideline is developed and implemented into practice (competency #17). Several of the students had heard about CPGs but never knew they should go through an appraisal process: They just assumed that if the guideline was published, it was trustworthy for practice.

Professor Sanchez invited the author of the CPG (Dr. Gomez, a pediatric nurse practitioner and recent DNP graduate) to their next class. Dr. Gomez discussed with the students how she identified the clinical issue in a pediatric medical center and began working with an EBP mentor and a team of interdisciplinary healthcare professionals through the EBP process. Dr. Gomez explained to the class that the process took 18 months and that many different disciplines were involved in the development of the CPG, including advisement from Professor Sanchez, her DNP advisor. Dr. Gomez shared with the class that the skill of critical appraisal was essential for the success of feeling confident in making the recommendations that she and her team published, and it was also very important to talk to parents of the patients that the CPG would impact. The students remembered that one of the quality ratings was related to the patients' views and preferences. The class realized that as master's-prepared nurses, they would be using CPGs to improve the outcomes in their practice setting. In addition, the class shared that they understood that to be able to develop a CPG, they would have to acquire a lot more knowledge in EBP—and that maybe a DNP might be in their future plans.

A REAL-WORLD EXAMPLE

TEACHING EBP COMPETENCIES IN CLINICAL SETTINGS

The first step of the EBP process is the spirit of inquiry. When stakeholders are involved, the spirit of inquiry naturally motivates the members through the work to be done—and, therefore, teaching EBP in a clinical setting is best done in an actual setting. An EBP mentor can guide, facilitate, demonstrate, and coach the members to reap the rewards of their efforts. The following is an example of where a group of staff nurses with an EBP mentor developed an EBP project, which started with their spirit of inquiry.

At this hospital, like all hospitals, there were multiple efforts to push the organization to achieve excellent patient outcomes and high patient satisfaction. Through one of the initiatives to promote effective rounding, a

continues

continued

technique was implemented on the advice of a consultant: to add "rounding sheets" in every patient's room. The intent was to provide a source of accountability for nursing staff to conduct their hourly rounds and provide evidence that someone had been in the room recently. Over time, the nurses and nursing assistants began to express extreme displeasure about the rounding sheets. It was not part of the permanent medical record and was perceived as busy work. Patients too frequently complained that staff would come into their room, sign the sheet, and leave.

Two medical-surgical units proposed a quality improvement (QI) pilot to remove the rounding sheets if the staff consistently documented rounding in the electronic health record (EHR) and their patient satisfaction scores for "responsiveness of staff" stayed better than the national benchmark. The pilot was successful (internal evidence), and the nurses asked whether the rounding sheets could permanently be removed. Nurse leadership responded that if a team of stakeholders (staff nurses) could find the evidence to support the decision, the annoying rounding sheets could be removed from practice. The Director of Patient Experience invited the EBP mentor and several nurses from the pilot units to create a team for the EBP project.

The EBP mentor had the opportunity to teach the team about the seven steps of the EBP process. She explained how their spirit of inquiry (Step #0 in EBP) had led to the QI pilot and now to engaging EBDM. The EBP mentor guided the team in Step #1 of the EBP process (write a PICOT question to direct the systematic search for external evidence). Two patient outcomes were chosen to be measured to indicate the effectiveness of rounding without the rounding sheets:

In adult med-surgical units in acute care (P), how does the use of rounding sheets (I) compared to no rounding sheets (C) affect patient satisfaction on HCAHPS scores on pain responsiveness (O1) and responsiveness of staff scores (O2) over 6 months (T)?

Step #2 in the EBP process began with the EBP mentor teaching the team about how to conduct a systematic search using databases such as CINAHL,

PubMed, and Cochrane. The team began with searching keywords from the PICOT question: patient satisfaction, patient rounding, and HCAHPS scores. The EBP mentor coached the staff nurses in the computer lab on basic search techniques, including the "search one AND search two" technique to find key evidence that included two shared concepts. The EBP mentor evaluated their success by reviewing screenshots of the team's search strategies from each database.

Step #3 of the EBP process included identifying the articles for rapid critical appraisal (RCA) to determine the keeper studies. The EBP mentor guided the team in using the RCA checklists that were appropriate for each study design. At the end of the RCA portion of critical appraisal, there were 17 keeper studies. The EBP mentor evaluated the success of the RCA process by reviewing the RCA checklists and associated rationale for why the team chose their answers to specific appraisal questions. The next step was to create an evaluation table with data from the 17 keeper studies. The EBP mentor assisted the team to extract data to complete the table and begin to consider synthesis of the evidence across studies. After the data were entered into the evaluation table, the EBP mentor guided the team to create two synthesis tables: a level of evidence (LOE) table and an outcomes table. In the LOE synthesis table, using the hierarchy of evidence for intervention questions, the team identified that there were eight Level III studies (nonrandomized trials); four Level V studies (systematic reviews of qualitative evidence; there were 63 studies evaluated within these four reviews); and five Level VI studies (descriptive, qualitative studies, or EBP implementation projects).

In the outcome synthesis table, the team described the 56 outcomes included in the studies, with 93% of the outcomes trending in the desired direction and 7% reported as no change in measured outcomes. Of the 17 studies, 9 reported statistically significant results. The EBP mentor suggested that the team add a column to the outcomes table that identified whether rounding sheets were part of the intervention strategy. Rounding sheets were not a factor in positive outcomes in 14 of the 17 keeper studies. The EBP mentor evaluated the team's learning through discussion of the

continues

continued

evaluation table and application of selected data extracted from the evaluation table to create the synthesis tables. The team's conclusion was the best evaluation of their cumulative learning about critical appraisal, and they recommended that purposeful rounding is needed to improve patient outcomes.

Step #4 in the EBP process involved presenting the evidence through the shared governance structure. As the EBP mentor guided the team through organizational change processes, the practice change to no longer require paper rounding sheets in the patients' rooms was approved by the Nursing Leadership Council as well as the hospital-wide Quality Council. The EBP mentor guided the team as they incorporated their clinical expertise into the presentation of this decision to the staff through telling stories of their experiences with rounding sheets and rounding without the sheets to provide context for the body of evidence within their organization. The team wanted to be intentional about including patient preferences and included in their stories some of the patients' complaints about the rounding sheets.

Step #5 included crafting an education plan about the change in practice that emphasized the body of evidence on effective patient rounding. Subsequent recommendations did not include paper rounding sheets. The EBP mentor recommended that patient satisfaction and pain responsiveness HCAHPS scores continue to be monitored and reported to staff for the next 6 months. Positive scores were the result, and the change in practice became the standard of care, which was the evaluation marker for a successful EBP process.

In Step #6, the EBP mentor suggested that the team construct a poster to describe their project experiences and outcomes that would be displayed at the annual hospital EBP & Research Conference. The team had no experience with poster design or presentation. The EBP mentor taught them about poster planning, execution, and delivery. The evaluation was complete when the EBP mentor observed the team confidently describing their work and its impact to the conference attendees. The EBP mentor queried the team about taking their work to a national conference, to which she received a resounding "Yes!"

SUMMARY

Evidence-based practice is well established as the foundation for best practice and nursing education. This approach to decision-making is expected for the 21st-century nurse. Curricula that address the EBP competencies have intentional innovation and purposeful integration of EBP in their foundations, content delivery methods, and evaluation strategies. Furthermore, a single EBP course is insufficient to bring about the required shift in how nurses think about their work—a shift to the EBP paradigm. Full curricular engagement is required to teach EBP competencies that offer sustainability of best practice because they become part of the DNA of every nurse.

REFERENCES

American Association of Colleges of Nursing (AACN). (2006). The essentials of doctoral education for advanced nursing practice. Retrieved from http://www.aacn.nche.edu/DNP/pdf/Essentials.pdf

American Association of Colleges of Nursing (AACN). (2008). The essentials of baccalaureate education for professional nursing practice. Retrieved from http://www.aacn.nche.edu/education-resources/baccessentials08.pdf

American Association of Colleges of Nursing (AACN). (2011). The essentials of master's education for advanced practice nursing. Washington, DC: American Association of Colleges of Nursing.

American Association of Colleges of Nursing (AACN). (2013). Competencies and curricular expectations for clinical nurse leader education and practice. Retrieved from http://www.aacn.nche.edu/cnl/CNL-Competencies-October-2013.pdf

American Association of Colleges of Nursing (AACN). (2015). The doctor of nursing practice: Current issues and clarifying recommendations. Retrieved from http://www.aacn.nche.edu/aacn-publications/white-papers/DNP-Implementation-TF-Report-8-15.pdf

American Nurses Credentialing Center (ANCC). (2014). ANCC Magnet Recognition Program®. Retrieved from http://www.nursecredentialing.org/magnet/

American Nurses Credentialing Center (ANCC). (2013). *2014 Magnet® application manual.* Silver Spring, MD: American Nurses Credentialing Center.

American Organization of Nurse Executives (AONE). (2015). Nurse executive competencies. Retrieved from http://www.aone.org/resources/nurse-leader-competencies.shtml

Brouwers, M., Kho, M. E., Browman, G. P., Burgers, J. S., Cluzeau, F., Feder, G., . . . Zitzelsberger, L. for the AGREE Next Steps Consortium. (2010). AGREE II: Advancing guideline development, reporting and evaluation in healthcare. *Canadian Medical Association Journal, 182*(18), e839–e842.

Centers for Medicare & Medicaid Services. (2014). Quarterly provider updates. Retrieved from http://www.cms.gov/Regulations-and-Guidance/Regulations-and-Policies/QuarterlyProviderUpdates/index.html

Ciliska, D. (2005). Educating for evidence-based practice. *Journal of Professional Nursing, 21*(6), 345–350.

Coomarasamy, A., & Khan, K. (2004). What is the evidence that postgraduate teaching in evidence-based medicine changes anything? A systematic review. *British Medical Journal, 329,* 1017–1022.

Epstein Educational Enterprises. (n.d.). What is the IF-AT? Retrieved from http://www.epsteineducation.com/home/about/default.aspx

Fineout-Overholt, E. (2015). Getting best outcomes: Paradigm and process matter. *Worldviews on Evidence-Based Nursing, 12*(4), 183–186.

Fineout-Overholt, E. (2013). Outcome evaluation for programs teaching EBP. In R. F. Levin & H. R. Feldman (Eds.), *Teaching evidence-based practice in nursing* (2nd ed., pp. 205–224). New York, NY: Springer.

Fineout-Overholt, E., & Johnston, L. (2005). Teaching EBP: A challenge for educators in the 21st century. *Worldviews on Evidence-Based Nursing, 2*(1), 37–39.

Fineout-Overholt, E., & Johnston, L. (2007). Evaluation: An essential step to the EBP process. *Worldviews on Evidence-Based Nursing, 4*(1), 54–59.

Fineout-Overholt, E., & Melnyk, B. M. (2006). *Organizational culture & readiness for system-wide integration of evidence-based practice.* Gilbert, AZ: ARCC Publishing.

Fineout-Overholt, E., & Stillwell, S. (2015). Asking compelling clinical questions. In B. M. Melnyk & E. Fineout-Overholt, *Evidence-based practice in nursing and healthcare: A guide to best practice* (3rd ed., pp. 25–39). Philadelphia, PA: Wolters Kluwer.

Fineout-Overholt, E., Stillwell, S. B., Williamson, K. M., Cox, J., & Robbins, R. (2015). Teaching evidence-based practice in academic settings. In B. M. Melnyk & E. Fineout-Overholt's *Evidence-based practice in nursing and healthcare: A guide to best practice* (3rd ed., pp. 330–362). Philadelphia, PA: Lippincott, Williams & Wilkins.

Greiner, A. C., & Knebel, E. (Eds.). (2003). *Health professions education: A bridge to quality.* Washington, DC: National Academies Press.

Halstead, J. (2007). *Nurse educator competencies: Creating an evidence-based practice for nurse educators.* Philadelphia, PA: National League for Nursing.

Institute of Medicine (IOM). (1999). To err is human: Building a safer health system. Washington, DC: National Academies Press.

Institute of Medicine (IOM). (2001). Crossing the quality chasm: A new health system for the 21st century. Washington, DC: National Academies Press.

Institute of Medicine (IOM). (2002). Educating health professionals to use informatics. Washington, DC: National Academies Press.

Institute of Medicine (IOM). (2010). A summary of the October 2009 forum on the future of nursing: Acute care. Washington, DC: National Academies Press.

Joint Commission. (2013). Revised requirements for the hospital accreditation program. Retrieved from http://www.jointcommission.org/assets/1/6/PrepublicationReport_CMS_HAP.pdf

Levin, R. F., Fineout-Overholt, E., Melnyk, B. M., Barnes, M., & Vetter, M. J. (2011). Fostering evidence-based practice to improve nurse and cost outcomes in a community health setting: A pilot test of the advancing research and clinical practice through close collaboration model. *Nursing Administration Quarterly, 35*(1), 21–33.

Melnyk, B. M., Fineout-Overholt, E., Gallagher-Ford, L., & Kaplan, L. (2012). The state of evidence-based practice in US nurses: Critical implications for nurse leaders and educators. *Journal of Nursing Administration, 42*(9), 410–417.

Melnyk, B. M., Fineout-Overholt, E., Giggleman, M., & Cruz, R. (2010). Correlates among cognitive beliefs, EBP implementation, organizational culture, cohesion and job satisfaction in evidence-based practice mentors from a community hospital system. *Nursing Outlook, 58*(6), 301–308.

Melnyk, B. M., Fineout-Overholt, E., Feinstein, N. F., Sadler, L. S., & Green-Hernandez, C. (2008). Nurse practitioner educators' perceived knowledge, beliefs, and teaching strategies regarding evidence-based practice: Implications for accelerating the integration of evidence-based practice into graduate programs. *Journal of Professional Nursing, 24*(1), 7–13.

Melnyk, B. M., Gallagher-Ford, L., Long, L. E., & Fineout-Overholt, E. (2014). The establishment of evidence-based practice competencies for practicing registered nurses and advanced practice nurses in real-world clinical settings: Proficiencies to improve healthcare quality, reliability, patient outcomes, and costs. *Worldviews on Evidence-Based Nursing, 11*(1), 5–15.

Michaelsen, L. K., & Sweet, M. (2011). Team-based learning. *New Directions for Teaching & Learning, 128,* 41–51. doi:10.1002/tl.467

Moch, S., Cronje, R., & Branson, J. (2010). Part 1: Undergraduate nursing evidence-based practice education: Envisioning the role of students. *Journal of Professional Nursing, 26*(1), 5–13.

National Association of Clinical Nurse Specialists. (2008). Clinical nurse specialists core competencies. Retrieved from http://www.nacns.org/docs/CNSCoreCompetenciesBroch.pdf

National League for Nursing (NLN). (2012). *Outcomes and competencies for graduates of practical/vocational, diploma, associate degree, baccalaureate, master's, practice doctorate, and research doctorate programs in nursing.* Philadelphia, PA: NLN.

National Organization of Nurse Practitioner Faculty (NONPF). (2012). Nurse practitioner core competencies. Retrieved from http://c.ymcdn.com/sites/www.nonpf.org/resource/resmgr/competencies/npcorecompetenciesfinal2012.pdf

Parmelee, D., Michaelsen, L. K., Cook, S., & Hudes, P. D. (2012). Team-based learning: A practical guide: AMEE Guide No. 65. *Medical Teacher, 34*(5), e275–e287. doi:10.3109/0142159X.2012.651179

Quality and Safety Education for Nurses (QSEN). (2007). Pre-licensure KSAS. Retrieved from http://qsen.org/competencies/pre-licensure-ksas/

Quality and Safety Education for Nurses (QSEN). (2009). Graduate KSAS. Retrieved from http://qsen.org/competencies/graduate-ksas/

Wallen, G. R., Mitchell, S. A., Melnyk, B. M., Fineout-Overholt, E., Miller-Davis, C., Yates, J., & Hastings, C. (2010). Implementing evidence-based practice: Effectiveness of a structured multifaceted mentorship programme. *Journal of Advanced Nursing, 66*(12), 2761–2771.

PART IV

APPENDIXES

In the appendixes, you find tools, such as the PICOT worksheet and a completed RCA checklist, that help you integrate the EBP competencies in your everyday practice.

There is also a handy glossary for when you come across an unfamiliar term.

Appendix A 279

Appendix B 283

Appendix C 287

Appendix D 293

Glossary 297

Index 309

PICOT WORKSHEET AND SEARCH STRATEGY DEVELOPMENT

PICOT Worksheet and Search Strategy Development

Define your question using PICOT: Patient, Intervention, Comparison, Outcome, Time (if applicable)

P atient/Population: _____

I ntervention: _____

C omparison: _____

O utcome: _____

T ime: _____

List the main topics, keywords or subject headings from your question that can be used to search:

OUTCOME	INTERVENTION	COMPARISON	POPULATION
_____	_____	_____	_____
_____	_____	_____	_____
_____	_____	_____	_____

Next, what criteria (limiters) do you need to include in your search? *This will help cut down the number of citations while making a decision about which to keep.*

Publication date _____   Gender _____   Language _____

Age _____   Publication type _____   Journal subset _____

What databases will you be searching?

____ Medline/PubMed   ____ Cochrane databases   ____ Professional Associations

____ CINAHL   ____ National Guideline Clearinghouse (US) ____ PsycINFO

____ TRIP Database   ____ Google Scholar/Google   ____ Other

STEP 1

OR keywords, topics, term, subject headings within *each* PICOT element (population, intervention, comparison, outcome, time)

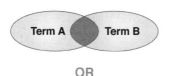

OR

Retrieves Term A, Term B, or
both Term A and Term B

STEP 2

AND to combine *all* PICOT elements

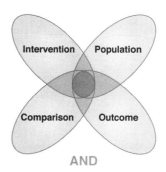

AND

Retrieves only citations which contain ALL
of the PICOT elements specified

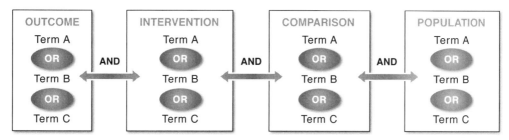

© Hartzell, 2015. May be reproduced without permission for educational purposes.

EXAMPLE OF A COMPLETED GENERAL APPRAISAL OVERVIEW (GAO)

General Appraisal Overview for All Study Designs

Date: Reviewer(s) name(s):

Article citation (APA): Darouiche, R. O., Wall, M. J., Itani, K., Otterson, M., Webb, A. L., Carrick, M. M., ... Berger, D. H. (2010). Chlorhexidine-alcohol versus povidone-iodine for surgical-site antisepsis. *New England Journal of Medicine, 362,* 18–26. doi: 10.1056/NEJMoa0810988

PICOT Question: In surgical patients (P), how does use of CHGA (I) compared to PVI (C) affect the SSI rate (O) post-operatively (T)?

Overview of Study

Purpose of Study: to determine the preoperative skin antisepsis that will reduce post-op infections.

Study Design: Randomized Controlled Trial (Level II)

Ethics Review Demonstrated (IRB noted):
The institutional review board at each hospital approved the study protocol, and written informed consent was obtained from all patients before enrollment (p. 19).

General Description of Study: A study of clean-contaminated adult surgical patients who had either CHGA or PI as their scrub/paint. Note to self: had to look up clean-contaminated—Medscape (http://www.medscape.org/viewarticle/448981_4) indicated *"A clean-contaminated surgical site is seen when the operative procedure enters into a colonized viscus or cavity of the body, but under elective and controlled circumstances." "The wound is judged to be clean when the operative procedure does not enter into a normally colonized viscus or lumen of the body."*

Setting was in 6 university-associated medical center. Notes to self: Since this was a university associated medical center, there were likely residents in these organizations performing surgery. The time frame was from 2004-2008...about 7 years ago...may be a little old, but is OK...also, it is interesting that the comparison was one agent with alcohol and one without...I wonder if that is a fair comparison? I wondered if the researchers really compared 3 agents? Or did the researchers confound the situation with the alcohol in one agent but not the other?

Time frame for completion outcome evaluation was 30 days—goal, reduce the rate of SSI. Note to self: The researchers randomized hospitals to CHGA, not individual patients to reduce the variability that may occur across hospitals.

Research Question(s) or Hypotheses:
1) Preoperative skin cleansing with CHGA is more protective against infection than PI.

Study Aims: The study aim was to test the hypothesis that chlorhexidine gluconate with alcohol (CHGA) is more protective than povidone iodine (PVI) regarding risk of postoperative surgical site infections (SSI).

General Appraisal Overview for All Study Designs

Sampling Technique, Sample Size, & Characteristics:
Sampling Technique—Primary author recruited hospitals to participate; within each randomized hospital, all 18 y/o and older surgical patients having clean-contaminated surgery were asked to participate (do not know by whom) (convenience sample); excluded allergy to CHGA, iodophors; evidence of infection at or close to op site; reported inability to stay in the study for 30 days
Sample Size: 849 (409 in CHGA; 440 in PI)

Major Variables Studied:
Independent Variable (IV): IV1-CHGA ; IV2- PI
Dependent (outcome) Variable(s) (DV): DV1- rate of SSI within 30 days; DV2—type of SSI

Statistical Analysis (include whether appropriate to answer research questions/hypothesis):
logistic regression to determine the odds of SSI happening in one group over another; spoke to using intention to treat analysis (good thing)

Conclusions: Authors concluded that in adult surgical patients with clean-contamination surgery, CHGA was better at reducing postoperative SSIs at the 30 day mark than PI...but the deal is that the PI didn't have alcohol, so the alcohol could be the real factor that is making the difference here...so wondering if it is a fair conclusion? Nonetheless, it is good to know that CHGA is better for patients than solely PI for preventing SSI and if there were ORs using only PI, they should change to CHGA—unless otherwise contraindicated.

NOTES for this GAO: This form is a working form in which clinicians have documented their thinking about this study as they recorded factual information. They have included notes to self that indicate their thinking and considered the TIPS provided to facilitate completion of the form.

EXAMPLE OF A COMPLETED RAPID CRITICAL APPRAISAL CHECKLIST WITH RATIONALE

Rapid Critical Appraisal Checklist for a Randomized Clinical Trial (RCT)—
Darouiche et al. (2010): Hypothesis: Average baseline rate of surgical-site infection
at the six participating hospitals was 14% after clean-contaminated surgery with
povidone–iodine skin preparation; we estimated that substituting chlorhexidine–
alcohol for povidone–iodine would reduce this rate to 7%.

1. Are the results of the study valid?	YES	NO	UNKNOWN
A. Were the subjects randomly assigned to the experimental and control groups?	YES		
B. Was random assignment concealed from the individuals who were first enrolling subjects into the study? The authors stratified their random assignment to hospitals; however, they did work toward concealment in that: "The operating surgeon became aware of which intervention had been assigned **only after** the patient was brought to the operating room." Note to self: The odd thing here is that stratifying the random assignment by hospital would make its concealment challenging after the first surgery—as the surgeon and OR staff would know which prep was being used in that hospital.	YES		
C. Were the subjects and providers blind to the study group? Both the patients and the site investigators who diagnosed surgical-site infection on the basis of criteria developed by the CDC9 remained *unaware of the group assignments*. Also, investigators who were *unaware of the patients' group assignments* assessed the seriousness of all adverse events and determined whether they were related to the study.	YES		
D. Were reasons given to explain why subjects did not complete the study? Yes, 36 patients were excluded from the per protocol analysis: 25 underwent clean rather than clean-contaminated surgery, 4 dropped out of the study 1 or 2 days after surgery, and 7 died before completion of the 30-day follow-up. Only the 4 who dropped out are of concern, but no reasons provided as to why.	YES		
E. Were the follow-up assessments conducted long enough to fully study the effects of the intervention? Follow-up was 30 days—long enough to detect an infection.	YES		
F. Were the subjects analyzed in the group to which they were randomly assigned? Intention to treat analysis was used.	YES		

1. Are the results of the study valid?	YES	NO	UNKNOWN
G. Was the control group appropriate? PVI was not alcohol-based and CHGA was; therefore alcohol could be confounder and may really be why the CHGA was a better prep. Since PVI comes in alcohol-based prep as well, the researcher should have had both as alcohol-based—this could influence the reliability of the study finding.		NO	
H. Were the instruments used to measure the outcomes valid and reliable? *Preoperative evaluation included a medical history taking, physical examination, and routine hematologic and blood chemical laboratory tests. The surgical site and the patient's vital signs were assessed at least once a day during hospitalization, on discharge, at the time of follow-up evaluation, and whenever surgical-site infection occurred. After discharge, the investigators called the patients once a week during the 30-day follow-up period and arranged for prompt clinical evaluation if infection was suspected. Whenever surgical-site infection was suspected or diagnosed, clinically relevant microbiologic samples were cultured. Investigators who were unaware of the patients' group assignments assessed the seriousness of all adverse events and determined whether they were related to the study.* (p. 20)—from this quote, it seems that the instruments are valid and reliable—but I don't know because there isn't enough information provided.			UNKNOWN
I. Were the subjects in each of the groups similar on demographic and baseline clinical variables? There were no significant differences on Table 1 (looked for a p value < 0.05).	YES		

continues

continued

2. What are the results?

A. How large is the intervention or treatment effect (NNT, NNH, effect size, level of significance)? The size of the intervention effect was indicated by the Relative Risk (RR) (the risk of the outcome in the exposed [intervention] group compared to the unexposed [comparison] group).

- The DV of *any surgical-site infection* had a RR of 0.59, p = 0.004.

- Note to self: This means that the risk of an infection for the CHGA patients was (1–.59 because 1 is 100% risk; therefore I subtracted the <1 risk for the exposed group .59 from 100% risk (1) to determine the decrease in risk in the exposed/intervention group) 41% less than the PVI patients.

- The DV Superficial incisional infection had a RR of 0.48, p= 0.008.

- Note to self: This means that the CHGA patients had (1–.48) 52% lower risk for a superficial infection than the PVI patients.

- The DV Deep incisional infection had a RR of 0.33, p= 0.05.

- Note to self: This means that the CHGA patients had a (1–.33) 67% lower risk for a deep incisional infection than the PVI patients.

B. How precise is the intervention or treatment effect? Note to self: The precision of the effect has to do with the confidence interval (CI).

For the statistically significant DVs:

- Any surgical-site infection had a 95% confidence interval of (0.41–0.85).

- Note to self: This is relatively narrow ensuring me as a clinician I can get somewhere close to the study findings. If it crossed 1, it would not be significant.

- Superficial incisional infection had a 95% confidence interval of (0.28–0.84).

- Note to self: This again is relatively narrow, but larger than DV1—still it ensures me as a clinician I can get somewhere close to the study findings. If it crossed 1, it would not be significant.

- Deep incisional infection had a 95% CI of (0.11–1.01).

- Note to self: This is a wider CI than my other significant findings, which makes me less confident in this finding. Also, the confidence interval crosses 1, which would technically be a non-significant finding, but the researchers indicate a *p* value equal to 0.05. I would be cautious with using this finding.

- Note to self: The other 2 DVs (findings) are not statistically significant and have a large 95% CI.

3. Will the results help me in caring for my patients?	YES	NO	UNKNOWN
A. Were all clinically important outcomes measured? • The researchers did include adverse reactions—none were statistically significant. However, cost was not provided. • Note to self: It seems reasonable that the cost of CHGA or PVI would not seem to be near the cost of one surgical site infection, but it would have been nice to have had those hard data documenting the costs. Also, it would have been a good thing to have the comparative costs across types of infections as they relate to the two surgical preps: CHGA and PVI.		NO	
B. What are the risks and benefits of the treatment? Risk of adverse events from both intervention and comparison were not greater than their benefit.			
C. Is the treatment feasible in my clinical setting? What are my patient's/family's values and expectations for the outcome that is trying to be prevented and the treatment itself?			NONE
Bottom-line Conclusion: This is a good study that offers information about whether or not CHGA compared to PVI decreases surgical site infection. The only question is whether they would get the same results with CHGA and PVI with alcohol?			

EVALUATION TABLE TEMPLATE

Citation: author(s), date of publication, title	Purpose of Study	Conceptual Framework	Design/ Method	Sample/Setting
First Author, Year, Article Title	The purpose is why the study was conducted? Consider that you could include the research question, hypothesis, or specific aims of the study.	Conceptual framework is the theoretical basis that guided the study.	Includes the research design that was used. Method means to describe briefly the study protocol (what they did).	Sample includes the number of participants, Sample characteristic e.g., (age, diagnosis) Setting means where study was conducted. Includes the attrition rate & why participants left the study?
Article 1				
Article 2				
Article 3	*add more rows as*	*needed to*	*accommodate*	*all studies*

Copyright Fineout-Overholt (2007)

The prompts offered for each column help you populate your table. Consider each prompt and enter the data requested into the evaluation table, but do not repeat the prompts in your table. When you have completed entry of all data from the keeper studies, remove the row with the prompts so that it is not confusing. Keeping all information succinct and clear (i.e., parsimony) is key. Do *not* use complete sentences. Use abbreviations and create your own unique legend to help readers read your table and readily see comparisons across studies. Keep your desired outcome in mind and *put only relevant information into your table.* Extraneous, unrelated content can confuse and take away from your relevant content and discovery.

Major Variables Studied and Their Definitions	Measurement of Major Variables	Data Analysis	Study Findings
Major variables are the: Independent variables Abbreviated: IV1 = IV2 = and the Dependent variables Abbreviated: DV =	Measurement of major variables refers to the dependent variable. Includes the scales used to measure the outcome variables (e.g., name of scale, author, information about reliability, such as Cronbach alphas).	In the Data Analysis column, list ONLY the name of statistics used to answer the clinical question (i.e., all statistics do not need to be put into the table)	Statistical findings or qualitative findings. IMPORTANT: for every statistical test you have in the data analysis column, you should have a finding. For example, if you put Mean Difference (MD) in the Data Analysis column, you should provide something like the following: MD IV1 & IV2 on DV = 13, p <.05.

GLOSSARY

Abstract: A summary of a publication that provides essential highlights to inform readers of the scope of a study or a presentation.

Adjacency searching: Helps the searcher retrieve words that are close to one another in a title or sentence. The words can be right next to each other or you may specify how many words come between each of the words you are looking for. Each database has a different method of executing this feature.

Applicability: Whether or not the findings of a study are appropriate for a particular patient situation or population.

Appraisal: Evaluating evidence for its worth to practice.

ARCC (Advancing Research and Clinical practice through close Collaboration) model: A framework to advance and sustain EBP in healthcare systems, which uses evidence-based practice mentors to facilitate EBP in point-of-care clinicians as the key strategy.

Article synopses: Summaries of the content of articles.

Bias: Deviation of results from the true values or the process that leads to such deviation.

Body of evidence: A comprehensive compilation of all the studies and reported projects that describe what we know about a clinical issue.

Boolean connector (operator) AND: The use of the Boolean operator AND allows the searcher to retrieve articles that contain all of the concepts that have been identified. It is the intersection of each of the different concepts. Using AND narrows the amount of articles retrieved.

Boolean connector (operator) OR: The use of the Boolean operator OR allows the searcher to retrieve articles that contain any of the concepts that have been identified. It is the union of similar concepts or synonyms. Using OR increases the amount of articles retrieved.

Case-control study: A study design that retrospectively compares characteristics of an individual who has a certain condition (e.g., smoker) with one who does not (e.g., a matched control or similar person who does not smoke); often conducted for the purpose of identifying variables that might predict the condition (e.g., stressful lifestyle, sodium intake).

Clinical inquiry: A consistently questioning attitude toward practice; an ongoing curiosity about best practices; inquisitiveness about the best evidence to guide clinical decision-making.

Clinical practice guideline: Systematically developed recommendations to assist clinicians and patients in making decisions about care that ideally have strong evidence to support the recommendations.

Cohort study: A study design that begins with the gathering of two groups of patients (the cohorts), one that received the exposure (e.g., to a disease) and one that did not, and then these groups are followed over time (prospective) to measure the development of different outcomes (diseases).

Competence: A concept that incorporates knowledge, skills, and attitudes referring to the ability to do something well.

Competency: An expected and measurable level of nursing performance that integrates knowledge, skills, and attitudes.

Competency blitz: Usually an annual event in which essential competencies are reviewed and where demonstration of competence is required.

Conceptual framework: Several interrelated statements that guide or direct a study or project; sometimes referred to as a *theoretical framework*.

Controlled vocabulary: A predetermined set of terms that help classify topics; also known as *subject headings* or *MeSH terms*.

Credibility: The accuracy of a qualitative study.

Critical appraisal: The process of evaluating a study for its worth (i.e., validity, reliability, and applicability to clinical practice).

Databases: Searchers use a bibliographic database to search the literature. This database collects and organizes (indexes) the literature in specific fields, such as medicine or nursing. Journal articles are primarily indexed, but dissertations, books, and conference proceedings may be indexed too.

Dependent variable: The variable or outcome that is influenced or caused by the independent variable.

EBP implementation: Putting into practice the best recommendations resulting from the seven steps of evidence-based practice designed to improve outcomes for a targeted patient population.

EBP mentor: Typically an advanced practice clinician with in-depth knowledge and skills in EBP, as well as in individual behavior and organizational change who guides others in EBP.

EBP paradigm: A worldview or set of beliefs, assumptions, and values that requires clinical decisions to be based on the amalgamation of existing well-done research, clinicians' expertise, including internal evidence, and patients' preferences and values. Each provider-patient encounter is unique and is allowed to flourish in a context of caring. The paradigm includes unique language and expected behaviors that lead to the outcome within the EBP paradigm, which is excellence in education, practice, and research.

EndNote: A proprietary reference manager: http://endnote.com/. A limited version is available for free: https://www.myendnoteweb.com.

Ethnography: A qualitative research design; the systematic study of a social group's culture through time spent combining participant observation and in-depth interviews in the informants' natural setting.

Evaluation table: A mechanism for transforming data from multiple studies into a matrix that allows for extraction of common and disparate data for synthesis.

Evidence-based clinical rounds: Rounds that are smaller in scope and more informal than grand rounds and are often conducted on patient units. They can be a very effective medium for disseminating evidence to a small group of colleagues to ultimately guide clinical practice changes.

Evidence-based decision-making (EBDM): Including best evidence in the decision-making process.

Evidence-based practice: A lifelong problem-solving approach to the way that healthcare is delivered that integrates the best evidence from high-quality studies with a clinician's expertise and a patient's preferences and values.

Evidence-based practice grand rounds: A mechanism for disseminating evidence to a large group of colleagues. Many hospitals and healthcare systems offer these as an opportunity to share the outcomes of EBP implementation or quality improvement projects and research studies as well as evidence-based recommendations for changes in practice based on a thorough review of a body of evidence. Grand rounds usually involve formal oral presentations followed by a question and answer interchange with colleagues.

Evidence-based practice implementation project: A project that is based upon the seven steps of evidence-based practice and implemented to improve outcomes for a targeted patient population.

Evidence-based practice seven-step process: A seven-step process used to deliver evidence-based healthcare, including: *Step 0.* Cultivate a spirit of inquiry within an EBP culture and environment; *Step 1.* Ask the burning clinical question in

PICOT format; *Step 2*. Search for and collect the most relevant best evidence; *Step 3*. Critically appraise the evidence (i.e., rapid critical appraisal, evaluation, and synthesis); *Step 4*. Integrate the best evidence with one's clinical expertise and patient preferences and values in making a practice decision or change; *Step 5*. Evaluate outcomes of the practice decision or change based on evidence; and *Step 6*. Disseminate the outcomes of the EBP decision or change.

Explode: The explode command in MEDLINE and CINAHL requests that the database search for the specified subject heading as well as more specific terms related to that subject heading.

External evidence: Data that is generated from rigorous research, which is intended to be generalized to other clinical settings to inform or improve practice.

Focus: The focus command restricts the subject heading to the primary focus of the article.

Full text: A copy of the entire article. Generally in PDF format, but occasionally it will be in HTML format.

General appraisal overview (GAO): A summary of the essential elements of a study, no matter what the study design (e.g., sample size, sample characteristics, setting).

Gestalt of study findings: Findings across multiple studies that meld into an understanding of best practices and lead to practice recommendations.

Grand rounds: A regularly scheduled meeting in which a clinical issue is presented through case examples and can include discussion of the progress of a patient from entry into a healthcare system through discharge.

Grey literature: External evidence that is generated primarily by organizations/associations such as government agencies, industry, or academia. It is not controlled by publishers and is often difficult to obtain.

Grounded theory: A systematic explanation of a situation-specific human experience/social phenomenon.

Hospital Consumer Assessment of Healthcare Providers and Systems (HCAHPS): A standardized survey instrument and data collection methodology for measuring patients' perspectives on hospital care.

Independent variable: The factor that is influencing the dependent variable or outcome; in experimental studies, it is the intervention or treatment.

Index(ing): The subject headings, controlled vocabulary, or MeSH terms assigned to an article to help a searcher retrieve the article.

Interlibrary loan: A service that a library provides to either borrow a book the library doesn't own or receive a copy of an article from a journal the library doesn't subscribe to.

Internal evidence: Data that is housed within a clinical practice setting from sources such as electronic health records, quality improvement or human resources departments, administration, and clinical systems or generated through quality improvement, outcomes management, or EBP implementation projects.

Interprofessional: Similar to transdisciplinary; meaning across different professions (e.g., nursing, medicine, pharmacy).

Journal club: A gathering of a small number of individuals for the purposes of incremental learning about a common topic of interest, sharing best evidence, and increasing EBP knowledge and skill levels, which can be conducted onsite or online.

Keeper studies: Studies retrieved in a systematic search that have been rapidly critically appraised and found to be relevant to the clinical question.

Keywords: A word or phrase that is not part of a database's controlled vocabulary (subject headings). Keywords can appear in the title or abstract of an article and are useful in determining what the subject headings are to reflect a particular topic. It is not always advisable to search using only keywords.

Knowledge broker: An individual in an organization whom others seek out when a question arises and needs to be answered.

Legend: A mechanism to provide the reader with the information that an abbreviation represents. Usually found at the bottom of a table or figure.

Levels of evidence: A ranking of evidence by the type of design or research methodology that most appropriately answers a specific question with the least amount of error and provides the most reliable findings; also called *hierarchies*.

Lived experience: Everyday experience as it is lived in the real world, not as it is conceptualized theoretically.

Logic operators: See Boolean operators; AND, OR.

Major concept: Within CINAHL, this allows the searcher to restrict the subject heading to the point of the article.

Mendeley: A free reference manager: http://www.mendeley.com.

Meta-analysis: A rigorous process of using quantitative methods to summarize the results of two or more studies to minimize bias. It is sometimes justified at the end of a systematic review, which identifies, appraises, and synthesizes studies to answer a specific question and draw conclusions about the data gathered. The purpose of the meta-analysis is to gain a summary statistic (i.e., a measure of a single effect) that represents the effect of the intervention across multiple studies.

Meta-synthesis: A holistic translation that is based on a comparative analysis of individual qualitative studies (interpretations) while retaining the essence of their unique contributions.

Monitor ongoing outcomes: Active gathering, evaluating, and reporting of clinical outcomes for the purpose of catching errors and correcting them.

National Guideline Clearinghouse: A public resource for evidence-based clinical practice guidelines (https://www.guideline.gov). It is an initiative of the Agency for Healthcare Research and Quality (AHRQ) with a mission to provide healthcare professionals, health plans, integrated delivery systems, and others an accessible mechanism for obtaining objective, detailed information on clinical practice guidelines and to further their dissemination, implementation, and use.

Outcome: The result of a healthcare intervention, treatment, or practice that can be quantified (e.g., number of complications, infection rate, length of stay in days).

Outcomes management: A process used by healthcare systems to define outcome targets, establish measurement methods, identify practices supported by evidence, and measure the impact associated with implementation of new interventions on healthcare quality.

Parsimony: A mechanism for being economical in words or in presentation of data in tabular form, usually by using abbreviations.

Patient decision support tool: Evidence-based information provided in a relatable and understandable format.

Peer review: An intentional process in which clinicians of like education and role review each other's work and provide constructive feedback to help improve the work.

Performance appraisal: A regularly scheduled evaluation of the performance of an employee and her/his impact on the work unit.

Performance expectation: A foundation for communicating about job performance that often includes: *results* (goods/services produced) and *actions and behaviors* (methods/means to create the product and behaviors/values demonstrated during the process).

Phenomenology: A qualitative research method of studying essences (i.e., meaning structures) perceived or grasped through descriptions of lived experience.

PICOT boxes: A creative strategy for promoting and collecting clinical questions. Simple boxes placed around a clinical area where clinicians can write down and submit clinical questions.

PICOT format: A process in which clinical questions are phrased in a manner to yield the most relevant information to guide an evidence search; P = Patient population; I = Intervention or issue of Interest; C = Comparison intervention or group; O = Outcome; T = Time.

PICOT question: A clinical question posed in a particular format to guide the search for evidence including the Patient population, Intervention or area of Interest, Comparison intervention or group, Outcome, and Time.

Pre-appraised literature: Publications that have already been appraised for the quality of the study methodology and reliability of its findings.

Process measures: Those variables or factors that influence outcomes. For example, a nursing action that is a process measure that may impact the rate of ventilator-associated pneumonia (the outcome of care) might include how many times a patient is turned in 24 hours.

Proximity searching: A method used to search for two or more words that appear within a certain number of words from each other. Proximity operators may use a letter (N or W) and a number or some databases use the term *adj* along with a number to indicate how many words can occur between the specified words.

PubMed: Freely available database that indexes the literature of medicine, nursing, and allied health. Available at http://www.pubmed.gov.

Quadruple Aim in Healthcare: A framework for optimizing healthcare that consists of: (1) improving the patient experience of care (including quality and satisfaction); (2) improving the health of populations; (3) reducing the per capita cost of healthcare; and (4) improving work life and decreasing burnout in clinicians.

Qualitative study: Research study designs used to develop in-depth understandings of people's experiences, beliefs, and motivations. It is primarily exploratory research that may be used to develop ideas or hypotheses for further investigation.

Quality improvement: Systematic and continuous actions that analyze existing data and lead to improvement in health services and the health outcomes of targeted patient groups.

Quantitative study: Research study designs where data is collected in numeric form and emphasizes precise measurement of variables.

Quasi-experimental studies: Research study designs that test the effects of an intervention or treatment but lack one or more characteristics of a true experiment (e.g., random assignment; a control or comparison group).

Randomized controlled trial: A research study design that is a true experiment and the strongest type of intervention study. Participants are randomly assigned to control or experimental groups. The experimental group receives an intervention or treatment and its impact is evaluated on one or more outcomes. It is the best design to establish cause and effect relationships between interventions and outcomes.

Rapid critical appraisal: A methodology for determining which studies found in a systematic search are relevant to the clinical question and worthy of keeping in the body of evidence.

Rapid critical appraisal (RCA) checklists: Tools that assist clinicians in evaluating validity, reliability, and applicability of a study in a time-efficient way.

Recommendation: A statement based on evidence synthesis indicating best practice and how it should be implemented and evaluated. Often recommendations lead to policy development and practice-change implementation.

Reference manager: Software that allows searchers to save and share citations they have retrieved. The citations that are collected can be easily edited, and new citations are continuously added.

RefWorks: A proprietary reference manager: http://www.refworks.com.

Reliability (of study findings): The replicability of study findings in practice; that is, if clinicians implement the findings in practice they should confidently expect the outcome found in the study.

"So-what" outcomes: Those outcomes that are important to the healthcare system, such as length of stay, post-operative complications, rehospitalization rates, and cost.

Stakeholder: A person or group that has an investment, share, or interest in something.

Strength of evidence: An overall assessment of the body of evidence that takes into account the methodology of the research study (study design), its quality, the balance of harms and benefits, and other factors that support clinical recommendations. Strong recommendations lead clinicians to confident action.

Subject headings: A predetermined set of terms that help classify topics; also known as *controlled vocabulary.*

Synthesis: Integrating the results of several studies to create an overall valuation of an entire body of evidence.

Systematic review: A summary of evidence that uses a rigorous process to identify, appraise, and synthesize studies to answer a specific clinical question and draw conclusions about the data gathered.

Transdisciplinary: Similar to interprofessional, meaning across different professions (e.g., nursing, medicine, pharmacy).

TRIP database: A clinical search engine that locates high-quality research evidence in healthcare. Available at https://www.tripdatabase.com/.

Triple Aim in Healthcare: A framework for optimizing healthcare that consists of: (1) improving the patient experience of care (including quality and satisfaction); (2) improving the health of populations; and (3) reducing the per capita cost of healthcare.

Truncation: A method used to search on the root of a word so that variations on the root will also be retrieved. It involves the use of a symbol, frequently an asterisk, being placed at the end of the root. For example, *increas** will also retrieve *increase, increased, increasing,* and *increasingly.*

Trustworthiness: The validity of a qualitative study.

Validity (of study findings): Whether or not researchers did a good job of using rigorous methodology to conduct a study and the influence of that rigor on the results of the study.

Yield: The number of citations that are retrieved by the search strategy.

Zotero: A free reference manager: http://www.zotero.org.

INDEX

A

academic medical center infrastructures, 211–222

Adult-Gerontology Acute Care Nurse Practitioner, MSN concentration, 267

advanced practice nurses (APNs), 11, 20

    assessments (of competencies)

        #1 (questions clinical practices), 42

        #2 (clinical problems using internal evidence), 47

        #3 (PICOT question formulation), 50

        #4 (searching external evidence), 67

        #5 (critical appraisal of pre-appraised evidence), 92–93

        #6 (critical appraisal of published research), 94–96

        #7 (synthesis of a body of evidence), 97–98

        #8 (collects practice data), 134

        #9 (evidence integration), 118–119

        #10 (practice change implementation), 119–120

        #11 (outcome evaluation), 135–136

        #12 (disseminating best practices), 177

        #13 (strategies to sustain EBP), 154

        #14 (searching external evidence), 71–72

        #15 (appraises pre-appraised evidence), 100–101

        #16 (internal/external evidence integration), 121–122

        #17 (transdisciplinary team leadership), 123

        #18 (internal evidence through OM), 136

        #19 (process measurement), 137

        #20 (evidence-based policies/procedures), 124

        #21 (external evidence generation), 138

        #22 (mentorships), 156

        #23 (sustaining EBP cultures), 157

        #24 (communicating best evidence), 178–179

    competencies, 25–27

    Delphi studies, 23–24

    job descriptions, 29

    journal clubs, 166

role of, 205–222
systematic approach to searching, 58–62
teaching examples, 267–269
advancement, CNS RBP competency, 212–216
affective commitment, 196
Agency for Healthcare Research and Quality (AHRQ), 166
AGREE II, 268
American Cancer Society, 71
American College of Chest Physicians, 57
American College of Gastroenterology (ACG), 73
American Journal of Nursing, 5, 96, 172
American Nurses Association (ANA), 21, 22, 196
American Organization of Nurse Executives, 145
AND operators, 59. *See also* searching
appraisal (critical), 77–106
evaluation, 86
group approach to, 89–106
pre-appraised evidence, 90–93, 98–101
process of, 81–89
published research studies, 93–96
rapid critical appraisals (RCAs), 83–86
recommendations, 88–90
synthesis, 87–88
ARCC model, 40, 151–153, 206
asking questions, templates, 51
assessments (of competencies)
#1 (questions clinical practice), 42
#2 (clinical problems using internal evidence), 47
#3 (clinical questions using PICOT), 50
#4 (systematic searches for external evidence), 67
#5 (critical appraisal of pre-appraised evidence), 92–93
#6 (critical appraisal of published research), 94–96
#7 (synthesis of a body of evidence), 97–98
#8 (collects practice data), 134
#9 (evidence integration), 118–119
#10 (practice change implementation), 119–120
#11 (outcome evaluation), 135–136

#12 (disseminating best practices), 177
#13 (strategies to sustain EBP), 154
#14 (exhaustive searches for external evidence), 71–72
#15 (relevant pre-appraised evidence), 100–101
#16 (internal/external evidence integration), 121–122
#17 (transdisciplinary team leadership), 123
#18 (internal evidence through OM), 136
#19 (process measurement), 137
#20 (evidence-based policies/procedures), 124
#21 (external evidence generation), 138
#22 (mentorships), 156
#23 (sustaining EBP cultures), 157
#24 (communicating best evidence), 178–179
policies, 228–229
Association of peri-Operative Registered Nurses (AORN), 71, 80
Association of Women's Health, 130
Associations for Professionals in Infection Control (APIC), 105
attributes of leadership, 147–151

B

behaviors, search strategies, 60–62
best evidence
inclusion of, 187
searching for, 55–74
body mass index (BMI), 179
body of evidence, evaluation of a, 96–101
Boolean operators, 59. *See also* searching
boxes, PICOT, 40
briefs for policy change, 176

C

calculating ROI, 195–198
catheter-associated urinary tract infections (CAUTIs), 4, 46
Center for Transdisciplinary Evidence-based Practice (CTEP), 21, 212

Centers for Disease Control and Prevention (CDC), 105

Centers for Medicare and Medicaid Services (CMS), 104

central line-associated bloodstream infection (CLABSI) rates, 46, 104

change
  briefs for policy, 176
  planning for, 112–113
  tools to guide process of, 114–124

checklists
  committee process, 236
  projects, 115–116
  rapid critical appraisals (RCAs), 14, 79, 83, 89, 93, 98, 103, 263, 271

chief nursing executives (CNEs), 147, 149

chief nursing officers (CNOs), 147, 149

chlorhexidine gluconate (CHGA), 78, 80

clinical expertise, 187

clinical inquiries, 33–53, 187
  cultures, 36–38
  definition of, 35–36

Clinical Ladder programs, 191–192, 220

clinical nurse specialists (CNSs), 206, 207–209, 267
  academic medical center infrastructures, 211–222
  competencies (EBP), 210–211
  mentorships, 209–210

clinical practice, 221

clinical settings, teaching EBP competencies in, 269–272

Clinical Standards and Practice Committee, 220

Cochrane Central Register of Controlled Trials, 4–5

Cochrane Database of Systematic Reviews, 4, 35, 130, 166

Cochrane Library, 56, 126

cognitive-behavioral therapy (CBT), 179

collaboration, 22, 201

colleagues, disseminating evidence to, 165–167

committees
  feedback, 24
  interprofessional education frameworks, 229–233
  membership changes, 235
  outcomes of processes, 236
  Patient/Family Care Policy Committee, 226–228, 236, 237–243
  policies/procedures, 193–194, 225–243

communication skills, 202

competence (EBP), 206

competencies (EBP)
  #1 (questions clinical practices), 38–45, 52–53, 265–266
  #2 (clinical problems using internal evidence), 46–47, 52–53, 265–266
  #3 (clinical questions using PICOT), 47–53, 265–266
  #4 (systematic searches for external evidence), 62–67, 72–74
  #5 (critical appraisal of pre-appraised evidence), 90–93, 104–106
  #6 (critical appraisal of published research), 93–96, 102–104
  #7 (synthesis of a body of evidence), 96–98, 102–104
  #8 (collects practice data), 134
  #9 (evidence integration), 117–119, 125–128
  #10 (practice change implementation), 119–120, 125–128
  #11 (outcome evaluation), 135–136, 139
  #12 (disseminating best practices), 176–177, 179–180
  #13 (strategies to sustain EBP), 153–154, 158–159
  #14 (exhaustive searches for external evidence), 67–74
  #15 (relevant pre-appraised evidence), 98–101, 102–104, 104–106, 140–141
  #16 (internal/external evidence integration), 120–122, 125–128
  #17 (transdisciplinary team leadership), 122–123, 125–128
  #18 (internal evidence through OM), 136, 140–141
  #19 (process measurement), 137, 140–141
  #20 (evidence-based policies/procedures), 123–124, 125–128
  #21 (external evidence generation), 138, 140–141

#22 (mentorships), 155-156, 158-159
#23 (sustaining EBP cultures), 156-157,
    158-159
#24 (communicating best evidence), 177-
    179, 179-180
advanced practice nurses (APNs), 25-27
clinical inquiries, 33-53
clinical nurse specialists (CNSs), 210-211
critical appraisal, 77-106
development of, 19-29
disseminating evidence, 163-180
educational program development,
    198-200
in healthcare settings, 185-203
implications for the use of, 28-29
importance of, 21-27
matching to existing standards, 249-261
measurements of, 186
outcomes evaluation, 129-141
policy/procedure committees, 225-243
practice leadership, 143-159
rationale for, 16
registered nurses (RNs), 25-27
role of advanced practice nurses (APNs),
    205-222
searching for best evidence, 55-74
teaching, 245-272
validation, 23
conceptual framework for healthcare, 9
consultation, 215-216
continuing professional development (CPD),
    196
Coordinating Council, 217
COPE (Creating Opportunities for Personal
    Empowerment), 7, 179, 180
costs, healthcare, 4
councils
    evidence-based practice (EBP), 154
    governance, 187, 192-193, 216-221, 263
    Nursing Leadership Council, 272
    Quality Council, 272
Creating Opportunities for Parent
    Empowerment (COPE) Program, 7, 179, 180
critical appraisal, 77-106
    evaluation, 86
    group approach to, 89-106

of pre-appraised evidence, 90-93, 98-101
process of, 81-89
of published research studies, 93-96
rapid critical appraisals (RCAs), 83-86
recommendations, 88-90
synthesis, 87-88
critical thinking skills, 202
cultures, 28
    clinical inquiries, 36-38
    evidence-based practice (EBP), 145-151
    sustaining, 153-154, 156-157
Cumulative Index to Nursing and Allied Health
    Literature (CINAHL), 4, 35, 56, 64, 73, 110,
    126, 130, 166

D

dashboards, 133
Database of Abstracts of Reviews of Effects
    (DARE), 5
deep vein thrombosis (DVT), 56
Delphi studies, 23-24, 201
development
    educational program, 198-200
    of evidence-based practice (EBP), 19-29
    of knowledge and skills, 231
    policies, 237-243
    professional, 221
    skills, 201-202
disseminating evidence, 163-180
    best practices, 176-177
    briefs for policy change, 176
    to colleagues, 165-167
    communications, 177-179
    importance of, 164-176
    lay/media publications, 175
    oral presentations at conferences, 167-169
    poster presentations, 169-170
    publications, 171-175
    strategies, 165
Doctor of Nursing Practice (DNP), 144, 207,
    267
domains, research, 215

E

EBP and Research Council, 5
EBP Project Planner, 114–115
education, 215
  clinical nurse specialists (CNSs), 207
  interprofessional education frameworks, 229–233
  opportunities for learning, 201
  policies, 228–229
  staff, 221
educational program development, 198–200
electronic health records (EHRs), 213, 270
emergency department (ED), 11, 51
environments, 28, 145–151
errors, reducing, 197–198
evaluation
  appraisal (critical), 86
  of a body of evidence, 96–98
  evaluation table templates, 293–295
  evidence-based decision-making (EBDM), 135–136
  outcomes, 15, 129–141
  performance, 29
  strategies, 262–264
events, sentinel, 197–198
evidence. *See also* evidence-based practice (EBP)
  collecting/searching, 13–14
  critical appraisal of, 14
  disseminating, 163–180
  external, 133
  hierarchy rating systems, 10
  integration, 15
  internal, 133
  intervention questions, 78–79
  levels-of-evidence (LOE), 80
  outcome evaluation, 15
  searching for best, 55–74
evidence-based decision-making (EBDM), 79, 81, 88–90, 246, 247
  mentorships, 154–155
  outcome evaluation, 135–136
  practice leadership, 143–159
  process measurements, 137
evidence-based knowledge and skills, 187

evidence-based practice (EBP)
  calculating ROI, 195–198
  clinical inquiries, 33–53
  competencies
    #1 (questions clinical practices), 38–45, 52–53, 265–266
    #2 (clinical problems using internal evidence), 46–47, 52–53, 265–266
    #3 (clinical questions using PICOT), 47–53, 265–266
    #4 (systematic searches for external evidence), 62–67, 72–74
    #5 (critical appraisal of pre-appraised evidence), 90–93, 104–106
    #6 (critical appraisal of published research), 93–96, 102–104
    #7 (synthesis of a body of evidence), 96–98, 102–104
    #8 (collects practice data), 134
    #9 (evidence integration), 117–119, 125–128
    #10 (practice change implementation), 119–120, 125–128
    #11 (outcome evaluation), 135–136, 139
    #12 (disseminating best practices), 176–177, 179–180
    #13 (strategies to sustain EBP), 153–154, 158–159
    #14 (exhaustive searches for external evidence), 67–74
    #15 (relevant pre-appraised evidence), 98–101, 102–104, 104–106, 140–141
    #16 (internal/external evidence integration), 120–122, 125–128
    #17 (transdisciplinary team leadership), 122–123, 125–128
    #18 (internal evidence through OM), 136, 140–141
    #19 (process measurement), 137, 140–141
    #20 (evidence-based policies/procedures), 123–124, 125–128
    #21 (external evidence generation), 138, 140–141
    #22 (mentorships), 155–156, 158–159
    #23 (sustaining EBP cultures), 156–157, 158–159

#24 (communicating best evidence),
177-179, 179-180
critical appraisal, 77-106
cultures, 145-151
definition of, 8-10
development of, 19-29
disseminating evidence, 163-180
educational program development, 198-
200
environments, 145-151
in healthcare settings, 185-203
implementations, 109-128
implications for the use of, 28-29
importance of, 21-27
matching to existing standards, 249-261
outcomes evaluation, 129-141
overview of, 3-16
policy/procedure committees, 225-243
Quadruple Aim in healthcare, 5-7
rationale for, 16
roles
    of advanced practice nurses (APNs),
        205-222
    of clinical nurse specialists (CNSs),
        207-209
searching for best evidence, 55-74
seven steps of, 10-16
sustaining, 143-159
teaching, 245-272
validation, 23
Evidence-Based Practice and Performance
Improvement Project Form, 57-58
evidence-based recommendations, 188
evidence-review manuscripts, 172
existing standards, matching EBP to, 249-261
external evidence, 25, 27, 34, 62, 67, 81, 86,
91, 98, 116, 130, 133, 138, 213

F

Fall Practice Problem Group (FPPG), 218
Fall Risk Stratification Wheel, 219
feedback, 23, 25, 35, 49, 50, 171, 174, 221, 241
    committees, 24
    immediate feedback assessment technique
        (IF-AT), 268
financial management, 195
frameworks, interprofessional education,
229-233

G

general appraisal overview (GAO), 83, 283-285
governance councils, 192-193, 216-221
GRADE leveling system, 82, 105
grand rounds, 166
grey literature, 71
groups, approach to appraisal (critical), 89-106
guidelines, 57, 165. *See also* National
    Guideline Clearinghouse
    Agency for Healthcare Research and Quality
        (AHRQ), 166
    Patient/Family Care Policy Committee, 236
    writing, 173, 174

H

HCAHPS scores, 272
Health Affairs, 176
healthcare
    calculating ROI, 195-198
    competencies (EBP) in settings, 185-203
    conceptual framework for, 9
    costs, 4
    EBP integration strategies, 186-192
    educational program development, 198-
        200
    examples of integration strategies, 202
    interrelationships, 230
    leadership role requirements, 194-195
    opportunities for learning, 201
    policy/procedure committees, 193-194
    Quadruple Aim in, 5-7
    shared governance councils, 192-193
    skill development, 201-202
    Triple Aim in, 5-6
Health System Nursing Quality, Research, EBP,
    and Education Department, 212
Healthy Lifestyles TEEN (Thinking, Emotions,
    Exercise, and Nutrition) Program, 179
hierarchy rating systems, evidence, 10
hospital-acquired infections (HAIs), 104

I

immediate feedback assessment technique (IF-AT), 268

implementations of EBP competencies, 109-128
- #1 (questions clinical practices), 39-42
- #2 (clinical problems using internal evidence), 46-47
- #3 (clinical questions using PICOT), 50
- #4 (systematic searches for external evidence), 62-66
- #5 (critical appraisal of pre-appraised evidence), 91-92
- #6 (critical appraisal of published research), 93-94
- #7 (synthesis of a body of evidence), 96-97
- #8 (collects practice data), 134
- #9 (evidence integration), 117-118
- #10 (practice change implementation), 119
- #11 (outcome evaluation), 135
- #12 (disseminating best practices), 176-177
- #13 (strategies to sustain EBP), 153-154
- #14 (exhaustive searches for external evidence), 67-71
- #15 (relevant pre-appraised evidence), 98-100
- #16 (internal/external evidence integration), 120-121
- #17 (transdisciplinary team leadership), 122
- #18 (internal evidence through OM), 136
- #19 (process measurement), 137
- #20 (evidence-based policies/procedures), 123-124
- #21 (external evidence generation), 138
- #22 (mentorships), 155
- #23 (sustaining EBP cultures), 156-157
- #24 (communicating best evidence), 177-178

informatics, 22

inquiries
- clinical, 33-53, 187
- cultures, 36-38
- definition of, 35-36
- spirit of, cultivating, 11-12

Institute of Medicine (IOM), 22, 59, 206, 228, 230

Institutional Review Board (IRB), 191

integration strategies, 186-192
- examples of, 202
- job descriptions, 187-189
- ladder programs, 191-192
- mentorships, 189-191
- mission statements, 187
- policies, 234-236

intensive care units (ICUs), 20, 139

internal evidence, 133
- outcome management (OM), 136

Interprofessional Education Collaborative Expert Panel, 230

interprofessional education frameworks, 229-233

interrelationships, 230

intervention questions, 78-79

Iowa model, 151

irritable bowel syndrome (IBS), 72

J-K

job descriptions, 29, 214-215
- integration strategies, 187-189
- mentorships, 44-45
- registered nurses (RNs), 43

job knowledge, 194

Johns Hopkins model, 151

Joint Commission on Accreditation of Healthcare Organizations, 197

journals
- *American Journal of Nursing*, 5, 96, 172
- clubs, 166
- *Health Affairs*, 176
- *Nursing Outlook*, 176
- *Worldviews on Evidence-Based Nursing*, 20, 139, 172

keeper studies, 14

keyword searching, 13, 56, 66, 281

L

ladder programs, 191–192, 220
lay publications, 175
leadership
    attributes of, 147–151
    expectations to meet EBP, 28–29
    practice, 143–159
    role requirements, 194–195
leveling systems, 81
    GRADE, 82, 105
level of evidence (LOE) tables, 271
levels-of-evidence (LOE), 80
libraries, Nationwide Children's Hospital
    (Columbus, Ohio), 231
Likert scales, 24
local conferences, 167–169
long-term acute care hospitals, 4

M

magazines, 175. *See also* publications
Magers, Tina, 4, 5
Magnet Forces (ANCC), 249
Magnet organizations, 226
management
    expectations to meet EBP, 28–29
    financial, 195
    leadership role requirements, 194–195
    outcomes management (OM), 132–133
    people, 195
manuscripts
    evidence-review, 172
    writing tips, 173
matching EBP to existing standards, 249–261
measurements
    of competencies, 186
    processes, 131–132, 137
media publications, 175
MEDLINE, 64, 73, 126, 130, 166
Melnyk, Bernadette, 172
mentorships, 24, 40, 269
    clinical nurse specialists (CNSs), 209–210
    evidence-based decision-making (EBDM),
        154–155
    feedback, 25

integration strategies, 189–191
job descriptions, 44–45
metered dose inhalers (MDIs), 11
metrics, patient satisfaction, 46
mission statements, 42, 187
Mississippi Baptist Health Systems, 4
models
    ARCC, 206. *See* ARCC model
    Iowa, 151
    Johns Hopkins, 151
Modified Early Warning Score (MEWS), 213

N

National Association of Clinical Nurse
    Specialists (NACNS), 207
National Association of School Nurses
    conference, 180
National Conference of State Legislatures, 168
national conferences, 167–169
National Database of Nursing Quality
    Indicators (NDNQI), 148
National Guideline Clearinghouse, vii, 57, 91,
    99, 105, 165, 166, 176, 268, 303
National Institute for Health and Care
    Excellence, 57
Nationwide Children's Hospital (Columbus,
    Ohio), 202, 226
    libraries, 231
    Patient/Family Care Policy Committee, 226–
        228, 236, 237–243
neonatal intensive care units (NICUs), 7, 130
nonjournal literature, 71
Nurse Educator, MSN concentration, 267
nurse practitioners (NPs), 226
nurses, 11, 20
    APNs. *See* advanced practice nurses (APNs)
    measurement of competencies, 186
    residency programs, 216
    retention, 196–197
    RNs. *See* registered nurses (RNs)
    sphere of influence (CNSs), 208–209
nursing
    missions, 42
    standards of nursing practice, 220–221

Nursing Administration, MSN concentration, 267
Nursing Leadership Council, 5, 272
Nursing Outlook, 176
Nursing Practice Council, 58
Nursing Quality Council, 5

O

Objective Structured Clinical Examination (OSCE), 67
Ohio State University
 College of Nursing, 21, 213, 229
 Health System (Columbus, Ohio), 202
 Wexner Medical Center (OSUWMC), 211
onboarding, 214
operating rooms (ORs), 78, 80
operators, Boolean, 59. *See also* searching
opportunities for learning, 201
oral presentations, 166, 167-169
organizational structures, realignment of, 212
Organization Infection Control Committee, 5
orientation, roles, 214
OR operators, 59. *See also* searching
outcome management (OM), 132-133, 136
outcomes
 of committee processes, 236
 defining, 131-132
 dissemination of, 15-16
 evaluation, 15, 129-141
 evidence-based decision-making (EBDM), 135-136
 sharing, 166
Ovid Clinical Queries, 5

P

Parents magazine, 175
Patient Care Council, 217
patient-centered care, 22
Patient/Family Care Policy Committee, 226-228, 236, 237-243
Patient Health Questionnaire (PHQ), 9, 158
patients
 interrelationships, 230

safety, 221
satisfaction metrics, 46
sphere of influence (CNSs), 208
voice, 187
Pediatric Nurse Practitioner, MSN concentration, 267
peer-reviewed journals, 173. *See also* journals; publications
people management, 195
performance evaluations, 29, 38
PICOT (Patient population, Intervention or Interest area, Comparison intervention or group, Outcome, and Time), 4, 10, 12-13, 35, 38, 102, 126, 139, 164
 boxes, 40
 clinical questions using, 47-53
 cognitive-behavioral therapy (CBT), 179
 in grand rounds, 167
 importance of, 231
 poster presentations, 169
 question templates, 51
 worksheets, 280
PICOT Worksheet and Search Strategy Development, 280
planning
 for change, 112-113
 EBP Project Planner, 114-115
policies
 assessments, 228-229
 briefs for policy change, 176
 committees, 193-194
 development, 237-243
 education, 228-229
 integration strategies, 234-236
 interprofessional education frameworks, 229-233
 Patient/Family Care Policy Committee, 226-228
poster presentations, 169-170
povidone iodine (PVI), 78, 80
PowerPoint presentations, 168
practice data, collection of, 134
practice leadership, 143-159
pre-appraised evidence, critical appraisal, 90-93, 98-101

presentations
    oral presentations, 167–169
    poster, 169–170
    PowerPoint, 168
Prevention magazine, 175
problem-solving skills, 202
procedures. *See also* policies
    committees, 193–194, 225–243
    integration strategies, 234–236
    interprofessional education frameworks,
       229–233
processes
    measurements, 131–132, 137
    outcomes of committee, 236
professional development, 221
Professional Development Council, 217
projects, checklists, 115–116
publications, 171–175
    lay, 175
    media, 175
published research studies, 93–96
PubMed, 5
pulmonary embolism (PE), 56

Q

Quadruple Aim in healthcare, 5–7
Quality and Safety Education for Nurses
    (QSEN), 22
Quality Council, 80, 272
quality improvement (QI), 22, 132–133, 168,
    221, 232, 270
questions
    in grand rounds, 167
    intervention, 78–79
    templates for, 51
    using PICOT. *See also* PICOT
       boxes, 40
       to formulate clinical, 47–53

R

randomized controlled trials (RCTs), 10, 103
rapid critical appraisals (RCAs), 14, 77, 79,
    83–86, 89, 271

checklists, 14, 79, 83, 89, 93, 98, 103, 263,
    271
    example of, 287–291
Rapid Critical Appraisal Checklist for a
    Randomized Clinical Trial (RCT), 288
rates
    catheter-associated urinary tract infections
       (CAUTIs), 4
    central line-associated bloodstream
       infection (CLABSI), 46, 104
    rehospitalization, 46
recommendations
    appraisal (critical), 88–90
    evidence-based, 188
regional conferences, 167–169
registered nurses (RNs), 11, 20, 139
    assessments (of competencies). *See also*
       competencies
       #1 (questions clinical practices), 42
       #2 (clinical problems using internal
          evidence), 47
       #3 (clinical questions using PICOT), 50
       #4 (systematic searches for external
          evidence), 67
       #5 (critical appraisal of pre-appraised
          evidence), 92–93
       #6 (critical appraisal of published
          research), 94–96
       #7 (synthesis of a body of evidence),
          97–98
       #8 (collects practice data), 134
       #9 (evidence integration), 118–119
       #10 (practice change implementation),
          119–120
       #11 (outcome evaluation), 135–136
       #12 (disseminating best practices), 177
       #13 (strategies to sustain EBP), 154
    Clinical Ladder programs, 191–192
    competencies, 25–27
    Delphi studies, 23–24
    job descriptions, 29, 43
    systematic approach to searching, 58–62
rehospitalization rates, 46
relationships, interrelationships, 230
research
    domains, 215

validation of EBP competencies, 23-27
Research, EBP, and Innovation Council, 217
residency programs (nurses), 216
retention of nurses, 196-197
return on investment (ROI), calculating, 195-198
Robert Wood Johnson Foundation, 229
roles
    of advanced practice nurses (APNs), 205-222
    of clinical nurse specialists (CNSs), 206, 207-209
    orientation, 214
    requirements, leadership, 194-195
Ross Heart Hospital (RHH), 212

S

sacred cows, 36, 37
safety, 22, 221
scales, Likert, 24
scores, HCAHPS, 272
searching
    for best evidence, 55-74
    keywords, 13, 56, 66
    strategies, 281
    systematic approach to, 58-62
sentinel events, 197-198
seven steps of EBP, 10-16
shared governance councils, 192-193, 216-221
Sigma Theta Tau International Research Congress (2015), 232
skills
    development, 201-202
    evidence-based knowledge and, 187
Society of Vascular Nursing, 58
staff education, 221
standards of nursing practice, 220-221
    matching EBP competencies to existing, 249-261
statements, mission, 42, 187
sticky learning, 247. *See also* education
strategies
    competencies
        #1 (questions clinical practice), 39-42
        #2 (clinical problems using internal evidence), 46-47
        #3 (clinical questions using PICOT), 50
        #4 (systematic searches for external evidence), 62-66
        #5 (critical appraisal of pre-appraised evidence), 91-92
        #6 (critical appraisal of published research), 93-94
        #7 (synthesis of a body of evidence), 96-97
        #8 (collects practice data), 134
        #9 (evidence integration), 117-118
        #10 (practice change implementation), 119
        #11 (outcome evaluation), 135
        #12 (disseminating best practices), 176-177
        #13 (strategies to sustain EBP), 153-154
        #14 (exhaustive searches for external evidence), 67-71
        #15 (relevant pre-appraised evidence), 98-100
        #16 (internal/external evidence integration), 120-121
        #17 (transdisciplinary team leadership), 122
        #18 (internal evidence through OM), 136
        #19 (process measurement), 137
        #20 (evidence-based policies/procedures), 123-124
        #21 (external evidence generation), 138
        #22 (mentorships), 155
        #23 (sustaining EBP cultures), 156-157
        #24 (communicating best evidence), 177-178
    disseminating evidence, 165
    evaluation, 262-264
    integration, 186-192. *See also* integration strategies
    searching, 58-62, 281
    teaching, 262-264
studies
    Delphi, 23-24, 201
    keeper, 14
surgical site infections (SSIs), 78
sustaining, 156-157
    evidence-based practice, 143-159

synthesis
    appraisal (critical), 87–88
    of a body of evidence, 96-98
    levels-of-evidence (LOE), 80
systematic approach to searching, 58–62
systems, sphere of influence (CNSs), 209

T

tables
    level of evidence (LOE), 271
    synthesis, 87–88
teaching. *See also* education
    evidence-based practice (EBP), 245–272
    examples of, 265–266
    strategies, 262–264
team-based learning (TBL), 267
team-readiness assurance test (tRAT), 268
teamwork, 22
technical skills, 201
templates, 232
    for asking questions, 51. *See also* PICOT
tools
    EBP Project Planner, 114–115
    to guide process of change, 114–124
traditions, 36. *See also* cultures
Triple Aim in healthcare, 5–6. *See also*
    Quadruple Aim in healthcare
Turning Research Into Practice (TRIP), 57

U–V

Unit Collaboration Council, 217
United States Preventive Services Task Force
    (USPSTF), 4, 158
Unit Leadership Councils (ULCs), 217
University Hospital (UH), 212
U.S. News & World Report, 226

validation of evidence-based practice (EBP), 23
ventilator-associated pneumonia (VAP), 145
voice, patient, 187

W–X–Y–Z

worksheets, PICOT, 280
Worldviews on Evidence-Based Nursing, 20,
    139, 172
Wound Practice Problem Group (WPPG), 218

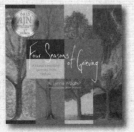
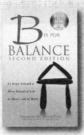
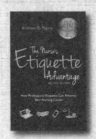
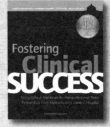
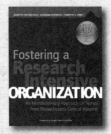
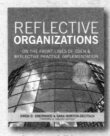
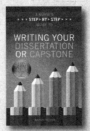

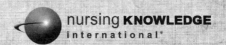

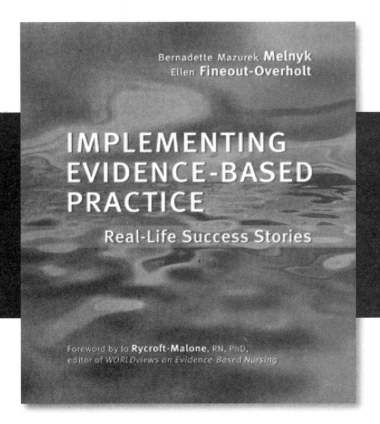
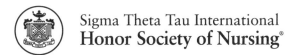
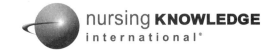

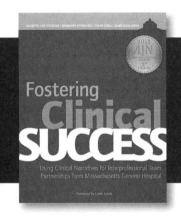
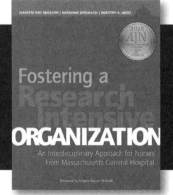
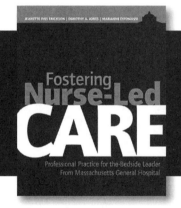

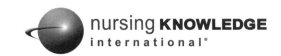